Fundamentals of VETERINARY ANATOMY

Fundamentals of VETERINARY ANATOMY

by
Jayant Aggarwal | Aniruddh Ahuja | Nishith Bhalla

Wordpen Academics
Publishing Science That Matter

ISBN: 978-93-6084-760-9 (Hardback)

Published by : **WORDPEN ACADEMICS**
4736/23, Ansari Road, Darya Ganj,
New Delhi – 110 002
Phone: +91-011-35004336
E-mail: info@wordpenacademics.com

***Printed at* : Replika Press Pvt. Ltd.**

Exclusive Distributor: ***Bio-Green Books, New Delhi***

PREFACE

"Fundamentals of Veterinary Anatomy" is a comprehensive and indispensable resource for students, educators, and practitioners in the field of veterinary medicine. This book is designed to provide a thorough understanding of the anatomical structures and systems of domesticated animals, laying the foundation for sound clinical practice, research, and education in veterinary anatomy.

Anatomy serves as the cornerstone of veterinary medicine, providing the structural framework upon which the principles of physiology, pathology, and clinical practice are built. A thorough knowledge of anatomy is essential for diagnosing and treating diseases, performing surgical procedures, and understanding the intricate relationships between form and function in animals.

As editors of this volume, we have endeavored to compile a wealth of knowledge from leading experts and educators in the field of veterinary anatomy. Through a blend of descriptive text, detailed illustrations, and interactive learning tools, this book covers a wide range of topics, including musculoskeletal, nervous, cardiovascular, respiratory, digestive, and urogenital systems, as well as comparative anatomy across different species.

Our overarching goal in presenting this book is to provide readers with a comprehensive and accessible resource that fosters a deeper understanding of veterinary anatomy and its clinical relevance. By emphasizing the importance of anatomical knowledge in veterinary education and practice, we aim to inspire a lifelong commitment to excellence and compassion in the care and treatment of animals.

We extend our sincere gratitude to all the contributors who have generously shared their expertise, experiences, and insights in the field of veterinary anatomy. It is our hope that this volume will serve as a valuable companion for students, educators, and practitioners alike, empowering them to excel in their pursuit of veterinary excellence and contribute to the health and well-being of animals worldwide.

Jayant Aggarwal | Aniruddh Ahuja | Nishith Bhalla

CONTENTS

1

INTRODUCTION

The term anatomy refers to the science that deals with the form and structure of animals. Physiology deals with the study of functions of the body or any of its parts. A thorough knowledge of the structure of an animal imparts a lot of information about the various functions it is capable of performing.

The course may be used as an introductory course to further studies; to assist you in recognising the normal, in order to determine the abnormal; to help you understand how to diagnose disease or determine if an animal has sustained an injury; to help understand the physical capabilities or limitations of particular species; to understand what happens in the nutrition and growth processes; and to assist you to get better performance from your animals. Anatomy (from Ancient Greek ἀνατομή (anatomḗ) 'dissection') is the branch of biology concerned with the study of the structure of organisms and their parts. Anatomy is a branch of natural science which deals with the structural organization of living things. It is an old science, having its beginnings in prehistoric times. Anatomy is inherently tied to developmental biology, embryology, comparative anatomy, evolutionary biology, and phylogeny, as these are the processes by which anatomy is generated, both over immediate and long-term timescales. Anatomy and physiology, which study the structure and function of organisms and their parts respectively, make a natural pair of related disciplines, and are often studied together. Human anatomy is one of the essential basic sciences that are applied in medicine.

The discipline of anatomy is divided into macroscopic and microscopic. Macroscopic anatomy, or gross anatomy, is the examination of an animal's body parts using unaided eyesight. Gross anatomy also includes the branch of superficial anatomy. Microscopic anatomy involves the use of optical instruments in the study of the tissues of various structures, known as histology, and also in the study of cells.

The history of anatomy is characterized by a progressive understanding of the functions of the organs and structures of the human body. Methods have also improved dramatically, advancing from the examination of animals by dissection of carcasses and cadavers (corpses) to 20th century medical imaging techniques including X-ray, ultrasound, and magnetic resonance imaging.

All vertebrates have a similar basic body plan and at some point in their lives, mostly in the embryonic stage, share the major chordate characteristics; a stiffening rod, the notochord; a dorsal hollow tube of nervous material, the neural tube; pharyngeal arches; and a tail posterior to the anus. The spinal cord is protected by the vertebral column and is above the notochord and the gastrointestinal tract is below it. Nervous tissue is derived from the ectoderm, connective tissues are derived from mesoderm, and gut is derived from the endoderm. At the posterior end is a tail which continues the spinal cord and vertebrae but not the gut. The mouth is found at the anterior end of the animal, and the anus at the base of the tail. The defining characteristic of a vertebrate is the vertebral column, formed in the development of the segmented series of vertebrae. In most vertebrates the notochord becomes the nucleus pulposus of the intervertebral discs. However, a few vertebrates, such as the sturgeon and the coelacanth retain the notochord into adulthood. Jawed vertebrates are typified by paired appendages, fins or legs, which may be secondarily lost. The limbs of vertebrates are considered to be homologous because the same underlying skeletal structure was inherited from their last common ancestor. This is one of the arguments put forward by Charles Darwin to support his theory of evolution.

Anatomy is the branch of biology concerned with the study of the structure of organisms and their parts. Here at Animal Corner we have compiled some of the most comprehensive diagrams and descriptions of all aspects of Animal anatomies so you can understand the specie you know and love. Interested in wolf paws and how those differ from domestic dogs? Our detailed approach allows you to research the key information you need for animals across the globe. Please browse the list below and learn the science behind the animal body.

HISTORY

Ancient

In 1600 BCE, the Edwin Smith Papyrus, an Ancient Egyptian medical text, described the heart, its vessels, liver, spleen, kidneys, hypothalamus, uterus and bladder, and showed the blood vessels diverging from the heart. The Ebers Papyrus (c. 1550 BCE) features a "treatise on the heart", with vessels carrying all the body's fluids to or from every member of the body.

Ancient Greek anatomy and physiology underwent great changes and advances throughout the early medieval world. Over time, this medical practice expanded by a continually developing understanding of the functions of organs and structures in the body. Phenomenal anatomical observations of the human body were made, which have contributed towards the understanding of the brain, eye, liver, reproductive organs and the nervous system.

The Hellenistic Egyptian city of Alexandria was the stepping-stone for Greek anatomy and physiology. Alexandria not only housed the biggest library for medical records and books of the liberal arts in the world during the time of the Greeks, but was also home to many medical practitioners and philosophers. Great patronage of the arts and sciences from the Ptolemy rulers helped raise Alexandria up, further rivalling the cultural and scientific achievements of other Greek states.

Some of the most striking advances in early anatomy and physiology took place in Hellenistic Alexandria. Two of the most famous anatomists and physiologists of the third century were Herophilus and Erasistratus. These two physicians helped pioneer human dissection for medical research. They also conducted vivisections on the cadavers of condemned criminals, which was considered taboo until the Renaissance—Herophilus was recognized as the first person to perform systematic dissections. Herophilus became known for his anatomical works making impressing contributions to many branches of anatomy and many other aspects of medicine. Some of the works included classifying the system of the pulse, the discovery that human arteries had thicker walls than veins, and that the atria were parts of the heart. Herophilus's knowledge of the human body has provided vital input towards understanding the brain, eye, liver, reproductive organs and nervous system, and characterizing the course of disease. Erasistratus accurately described the structure of the brain, including the cavities and membranes, and made a distinction between its cerebrum and cerebellum During his study in Alexandria, Erasistratus was particularly concerned with studies of the circulatory and nervous systems. He was able to distinguish the sensory and the motor nerves in the human body and believed that air entered the lungs and heart, which was then carried throughout the body. His distinction between the arteries and veins—the arteries carrying the air through the body, while the veins carried the blood from the heart was a great anatomical discovery. Erasistratus was also responsible for naming and describing the function of the epiglottis and the valves of the heart, including the tricuspid. During the third century, Greek physicians were able to differentiate nerves from blood vessels and tendons and to realize that the nerves convey neural impulses. It was Herophilus who made the point that damage to motor nerves induced paralysis. Herophilus named the meninges and ventricles in the brain, appreciated the division between cerebellum and cerebrum and recognized that the brain was the "seat of intellect" and not a "cooling chamber" as propounded by Aristotle Herophilus is also credited with describing the optic, oculomotor, motor division of the trigeminal, facial, vestibulocochlear and hypoglossal nerves.

Great feats were made during the third century BCE in both the digestive and reproductive systems. Herophilus was able to discover and describe not only the salivary glands, but the small intestine and liver. He showed that the uterus is a hollow organ and described the ovaries and uterine tubes. He recognized that spermatozoa were produced by the testes and was the first to identify the prostate gland.

The anatomy of the muscles and skeleton is described in the Hippocratic Corpus, an Ancient Greek medical work written by unknown authors. Aristotle described vertebrate anatomy based on animal dissection. Praxagoras identified the difference between arteries and veins. Also in the 4th century BCE, Herophilos and Erasistratus produced more accurate anatomical descriptions based on vivisection of criminals in Alexandria during the Ptolemaic dynasty. In the 2nd century, Galen of Pergamum, an anatomist, clinician, writer and philosopher, wrote the final and highly influential anatomy treatise of ancient times. He compiled existing knowledge and studied anatomy through dissection of animals. He was one of the first experimental physiologists through his vivisection experiments on animals. Galen's drawings, based mostly on dog anatomy, became effectively the only anatomical textbook for the next thousand years. His work was known to Renaissance doctors only through Islamic Golden Age medicine until it was translated from the Greek some time in the 15th century.

Medieval to early modern

Anatomy developed little from classical times until the sixteenth century; as the historian Marie Boas writes, "Progress in anatomy before the sixteenth century is as mysteriously slow as its development after 1500 is startlingly rapid". :120–121 Between 1275 and 1326, the anatomists Mondino de Luzzi, Alessandro Achillini and Antonio Benivieni at Bologna carried out the first systematic human dissections since ancient times. Mondino's Anatomy of 1316 was the first textbook in the medieval rediscovery of human anatomy. It describes the body in the order followed in Mondino's dissections, starting with the abdomen, then the thorax, then the head and limbs. It was the standard anatomy textbook for the next century.

Leonardo da Vinci (1452–1519) was trained in anatomy by Andrea del Verrocchio. He made use of his anatomical knowledge in his artwork, making many sketches of skeletal structures, muscles and organs of humans and other vertebrates that he dissected.

Andreas Vesalius (1514–1564), professor of anatomy at the University of Padua, is considered the founder of modern human anatomy. Originally from Brabant, Vesalius published the influential book De humani corporis fabrica ("the structure of the human body"), a large format book in seven volumes, in 1543. The accurate and intricately detailed illustrations, often in allegorical poses against Italianate landscapes, are thought to have been made by the artist Jan van Calcar, a pupil of Titian.

In England, anatomy was the subject of the first public lectures given in any science; these were given by the Company of Barbers and Surgeons in the 16th century, joined in 1583 by the Lumleian lectures in surgery at the Royal College of Physicians.

Late modern

In the United States, medical schools began to be set up towards the end of the 18th century. Classes in anatomy needed a continual stream of cadavers for dissection and these were difficult to obtain. Philadelphia, Baltimore and New York were all renowned for body snatching activity as criminals raided graveyards at night, removing newly buried corpses from their coffins. A similar problem existed in Britain where demand for bodies became so great that grave-raiding and even anatomy murder were practised to obtain cadavers. Some graveyards were in consequence protected with watchtowers. The practice was halted in Britain by the Anatomy Act of 1832, while in the United States, similar legislation was enacted after the physician William S. Forbes of Jefferson Medical College was found guilty in 1882 of "complicity with resurrectionists in the despoliation of graves in Lebanon Cemetery".

The teaching of anatomy in Britain was transformed by Sir John Struthers, Regius Professor of Anatomy at the University of Aberdeen from 1863 to 1889. He was responsible for setting up the system of three years of "pre-clinical" academic teaching in the sciences underlying medicine, including especially anatomy. This system lasted until the reform of medical training in 1993 and 2003. As well as teaching, he collected many vertebrate skeletons for his museum of comparative anatomy, published over 70 research papers, and became famous for his public dissection of the Tay Whale. From 1822 the Royal College of Surgeons regulated the teaching of anatomy in medical schools. Medical museums provided examples in comparative anatomy, and were often used in teaching. Ignaz Semmelweis investigated puerperal fever and he discovered how it was caused. He noticed that the frequently fatal fever occurred more often in mothers examined by medical students than by midwives. The students went from the dissecting room to the hospital ward and examined women in childbirth. Semmelweis showed that when the trainees washed their hands in chlorinated lime before each clinical examination, the incidence of puerperal fever among the mothers could be reduced dramatically.

Before the modern medical era, the main means for studying the internal structures of the body were dissection of the dead and inspection, palpation and auscultation of the living. It was the advent of microscopy that opened up an understanding of the building blocks that constituted living tissues. Technical advances in the development of achromatic lenses increased the resolving power of the microscope and around 1839, Matthias Jakob Schleiden and Theodor Schwann identified that cells were the fundamental unit of organization of all living things. Study of small structures involved passing light through them and the microtome was invented to provide sufficiently thin slices of tissue to examine. Staining techniques using artificial dyes were established to help distinguish between different types of tissue. Advances in the fields of histology and cytology began in the late 19th century along with advances in surgical techniques allowing for the painless and safe removal of biopsy specimens. The invention of the electron microscope brought a great advance in resolution power and allowed research into the ultrastructure of cells and the organelles and other structures within them. About the same time, in the 1950s, the use of X-ray diffraction for studying the crystal structures of proteins, nucleic acids and other biological molecules gave rise to a new field of molecular anatomy.

Equally important advances have occurred in non-invasive techniques for examining the interior structures of the body. X-rays can be passed through the body and used in medical radiography and fluoroscopy to differentiate interior structures that have varying degrees of opaqueness. Magnetic resonance imaging, computed tomography, and ultrasound imaging have all enabled examination of internal structures in unprecedented detail to a degree far beyond the imagination of earlier generations.

WOLF ANATOMY

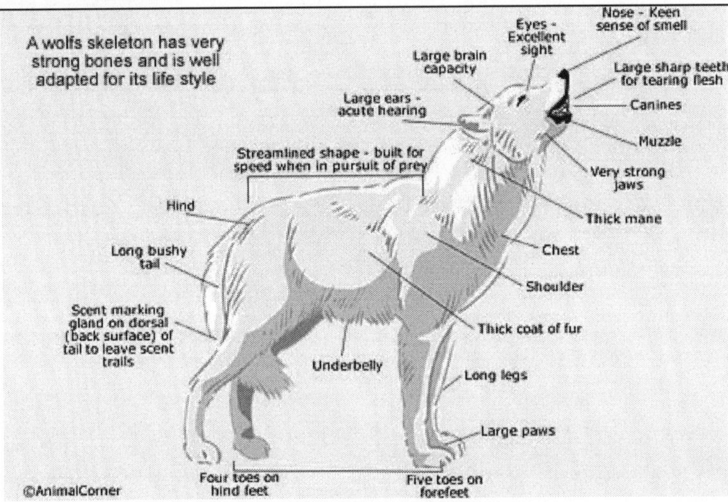

Fig 1.1

Muzzle – A wolf has two hundred million smelling cells inside its nose and can smell 100 times better than a human being. A wolf has 42 teeth including four canines. Wolves use their sharp teeth to wound, grab and kill its prey. Wolves use their back teeth to crush the bones and make the meat into smaller pieces and they use the small front teeth to nibble and pull at the skin. A wolf has a very rough tongue which is used for cleaning the meat off of the bones.

Eyes and Nose – Wolves move their ears from side to side to determine where a sound is coming from. Wolves have excellent eye sight, a keen sense of smell and acute hearing. Wolves can see and smell a deer from a great distance.

Body – A wolfs body is strong and powerful which enables it to kill large prey such as deer and elk.

Fur – The wolf has two layers of fur. On top is a longer course fur used as guard hairs which keeps the wolf dry. The other is short under fur that keeps it warm.

Legs and Feet – Wolves toes spread apart when they step in the snow so they do not sink. Wolves walk and run on their toes. It makes their legs longer and nimble so they can run with speed and catch fast prey. Wolves have four toes on their hind feet and five toes on their fore feet.

Tails – Wolves use their tails to communicate. For example, the tails position and the state of its hair send specific messages. Wolves also have a scent gland on the back surface of their tails which they use to scent-mark territory.

Skeleton – The skeleton of the wolf is well adapted to its lifestyle. Their bones need to be strong, for power in bringing down large prey such as caribou, deer, elks or moose. The narrow collarbones, interlocked foreleg bones and specially adapted wrist-bones give the wolf streamlining, strength and speed. The radius and ulna bones are 'locked' in position. This inability to rotate the forelimbs gives superb stability when running.

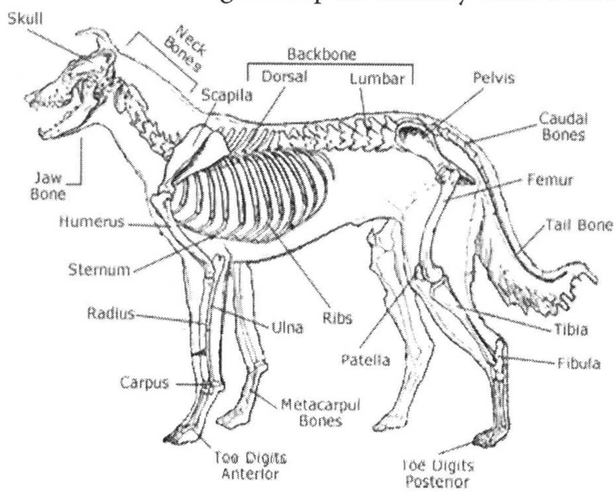

Fig 1.2

Long Skull – Wolves have long skulls which is a typical carnivore skull, housing extensive and strong cheek muscles, necessary for holding onto prey, killing and consuming.

Large Brain Capacity – Skull capacity allows adequate space for an advanced cerebral cortex (brain) necessary for coordinating group social activity.

Wolf Paws

Wolf paws are able to tread easily on a wide variety of terrains, especially snow. There is a slight webbing between each toe, which allows them to move over snow more easily. Wolves are digitigrades (an animal that stands or walks on its digits, or toes) and with the relative largeness of their feet, helps them to distribute their weight evenly on snowy surfaces. The front paws are larger than the hind paws and have a fifth digit, the dew claw, which is absent on their hind paws. A dew claw is a vestigial digit of the paw which grows higher on the leg so that when the animal is standing, it does not make contact with the ground.

Bristled hairs and blunt claws help wolves to grip on slippery surfaces, and special blood vessels prevent their paw pads from freezing. Scent glands located between a wolfs toes leave trace chemical markers behind, helping the wolf to effectively navigate over large areas while keeping others informed of its whereabouts. Unlike dogs and coyotes, wolves lack sweat glands on their paw pads.

Wolf Fur

Wolves have bulky coats consisting of two layers. Their first layer is made up of tough guard hairs that repel water and dirt. Their second layer is a dense, water-resistant undercoat that insulates the wolf and keeps it warm. Their undercoat is shed in the form of large tufts of fur in late spring or early summer (with yearly variations).

A wolf will often rub against objects such as rocks and branches to encourage the loose fur to fall out. Their undercoat is usually grey regardless of the outer coats appearance. Wolves have distinct winter and summer pelages (the hair or fur that covers the animal) that alternate in spring and autumn. Female wolves tend to keep their winter coats further into the spring than male wolves. North American wolves typically have longer, silkier fur than their Eurasian relatives.

The color of the wolfs fur varies greatly, from grey to grey-brown, to white, red, brown and black. These colors tend to mix in many populations to form predominantly blended individuals, though it is not uncommon for an individual or an entire population of wolves to be entirely one color (usually all black or all white). A multicolor coat lacks any clear pattern and tends to be lighter on the wolfs undersides. A wolfs fur color sometimes corresponds with a wolf populations environment, for example, all-white wolves are much more common in areas with snow cover. Aging wolves acquire a greyish tint in their coats. The Grey Wolf and the Red Wolf tend to have interspersed flicks of yellowish coloring appearing through their base color.

At birth, wolf pups tend to have darker fur and their eyes have blue irises that will change to a yellow-gold or orange color when the pups are between 8 and 16 weeks old. Though extremely unusual, it is possible for an adult wolf to retain its blue-colored irises.

How Wolves Differ From Dogs

A wolfs long, powerful muzzles help distinguish them from other canids, particularly coyotes and golden jackals, which have more narrow, pointed muzzles. Wolves differ from domestic dogs as they have a comparatively larger brain capacity. Larger paw size, yellow eyes, longer legs and bigger teeth further distinguish adult wolves from other canids, especially dogs. Also, precaudal glands at the base of the tail are present in wolves, however, not in dogs.

Dog Anatomy

Dogs grow in various sizes and shapes.

- The Greyhound is the 'Fastest Dog on Earth' and can run 45 miles per hour for short periods of time.

- The Irish Wolfhound is the largest dog standing 28 – 32 inches and weighing between 90 – 150 pounds. Irish Wolfhounds make excellent companions, however, their life expectancy is somewhat shorter than most dogs and is between 6 – 8 years.
- The Great Dane is the tallest dog standing 30 – 34 inches and weighing 120 – 200 pounds. These too have a short life expectancy and the average age is under 10 years although some can live 12 – 13 years. The Great Dane originates from Germany.
- The Chihuahua is the smallest dog standing at only 5 inches tall and weighing 2 – 6 pounds. Chihuahuas can live until they are 15 years old.
- The St. Bernard is the heaviest dog. They are very strong, muscular dogs with powerful heads, however, they are extremely gentle and friendly dogs and very tolerant of children. They stand around 26 – 28 inches and can weigh between 150 – 210 pounds.
- The worlds oldest dog was an Australian cattle-dog named Bluey who lived to the age of 29 years and 5 months.

Other breeds range in different sizes and weights between the above.

Below is a diagram of a dogs anatomy:

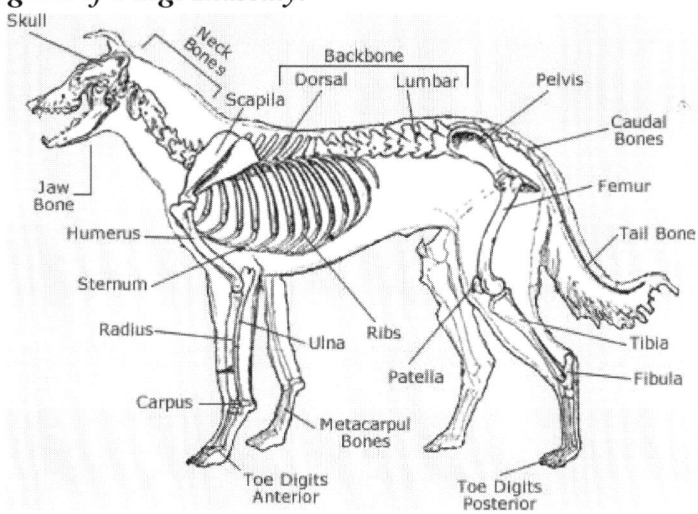

Fig 1.3

The coat of a dog varies in colors ranging from all black, brown, beige and white to others being of a mix with light or dark markings and colorations on different parts of their bodies and faces.

Their fur ranges from short, smooth fur to long shaggy fur to soft and fluffy to hard and coarse. The shape of a dog is determined by three structures, head, body and legs.

Short smooth fur Long fluffy fur

Shaggy fur Short soft fur

The shape of these structures vary greatly in the same way as their colors and hair characteristics. The two most common head shapes for a dog are a narrow skull with a long face, such as a German Shepherd and a short skull with a short face, such as a pug dog There are many variations to these shapes in between.

Dogs have 42 teeth. Six pairs of sharp incisor teeth are in front of the mouth, flanked by two pairs of large canine ('dog') teeth. The other teeth are premolars and molars. The incisors and the canines are very important because the dog bites and tears at its food with these teeth.

Dogs have fairly thin tongues which are used mainly for guiding food to the throat, for licking the coat clean, and for perspiration. When a dog is overheated, it cools off by hanging its tongue out and panting. As it pants, the evaporation of perspiration from its tongue cools the animal. The dog also sweats through the pads on its paws and very slighty through its skin.

Dogs ears either stick up or hang down. Dogs have extremely sensitive hearing and can hear far more high frequencies than human ears. This is why they respond to silent whistles.

A dog has three eyelids on each eye, the main upper and lower lids and a third lid hidden between them in the inner corner of the eye. The third eyelid can sweep across the transparent cornea of the eye and clean it like a windshield wiper.

The body of a dog contains most of its vital organs. The heart, lungs, stomach, and intestines are located there. So too are its genitals, kidneys and bladder. A dog has 13 ribs in its chest which wrap around the heart and lungs. Since these organs influence the animals speed and stamina, chest size can be an indication of these traits.

All dogs have 27 bones from the skull to the point where the tail begins. The number of tailbones, however and therefore the length of the tail, varies from breed to breed.

The front legs of a dog are called the 'forelegs' and the back legs are called the 'hindlegs'. On each paw, they have 5 toes, however, one of these toes of called the 'dewclaw' and is too high up to be of any use. The paw has cushiony pads for each toe and 2 larger pads further up the paw. Dogs perspire (sweat) through their pads.

A dogs heart beats between 70 and 120 times per minute, compared to a humans 70 – 80 beats per minute. Dogs take between 10 and 30 breathes every minute. Dogs have a visual range of 250 degrees compared to the human range of 180 degrees. A dogs temperature is between 100.2 and 102.8 degrees Fahrenheit. The average lifespan of a dog ranges from 12 – 14 years. Each one dog year is equivalent to 7 human years.

COW ANATOMY

Below is a diagram of the anatomy of a cow

As you can see, there are many parts to a cow.

Cows vary in all different colors, some are brown, tanned, white, black, brown-white patched or black-white patched. In a female cow, milk is produced in the udders and extracted from the teats. A Cows udder has four compartments with one teat hanging from each.

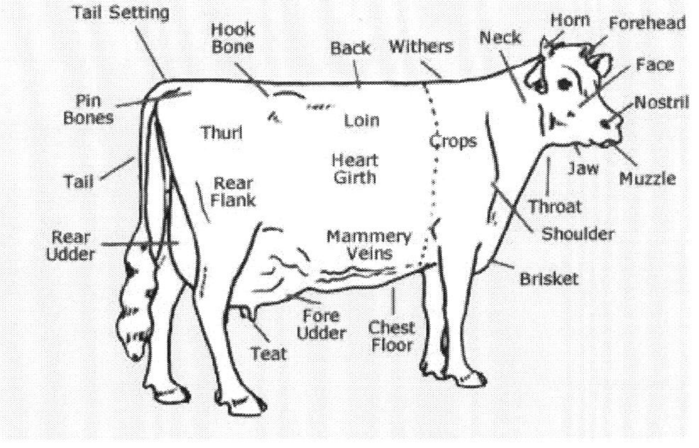

Fig. 1.4

Tiny Cells remove water and nutrients from the blood and convert it into milk. The milk forms into droplets and drips into a cistern which holds the milk. If the cows teat is squeezed, it produces a squirt of milk and is either saved in tanks or feeds a suckling calf.

A cows mouth is adapted for grazing, the top part of the mouth is a hard pad and the bottom part a row of flat-topped teeth. Cows have 32 teeth in all, 8 incisors on the bottom part and 6 molars on the top and bottom parts on each side.

The cow tears grass from the field and grinds it between the two mouth parts.

A cows ears are very flexible and can turn in any direction. They are especially used to hear any signs of danger from many directions.

Cows have long tails which they use to waft insects of them.

Bulls have horns, although some female cows have small horns too. Bulls horns are made out of similar material to our fingernails called 'Keratin'. Bulls horns can be removed without causing the cow any discomfort.

Diet

Cows are herbivores which means they do not eat meat, only plants, grass and cereal. Cows are ruminant animals which means they have more than one stomach.

Cows have a four part stomach, each part used for a different process.

Cows swallow their food without chewing it too much at first. Cows later regurgitate a 'cud' which is then chewed well and swallowed.

The Anatomy of a Cows Stomach

Inside a cows stomach region, there are 4 digestive departments:

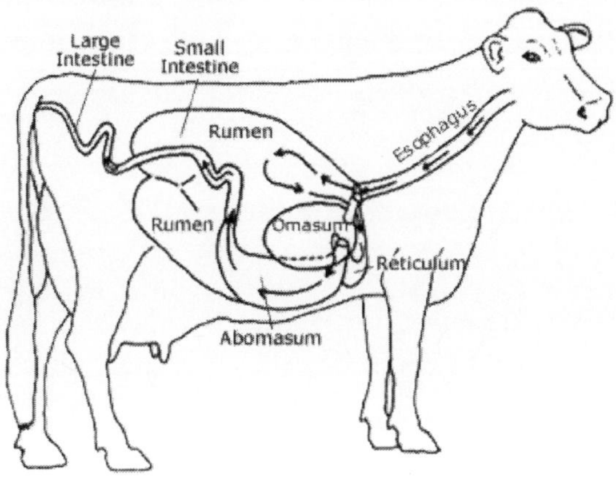

Fig 1.5

1. The Rumen – this is the largest part and holds upto 50 gallons of partially digested food. This is where the 'cud' comes from. Good bacteria in the Rumen helps soften and digest the cows food and provides protein for the cow.

2. The Recticulum – this part of the stomach is called the 'hardware' stomach. This is because if the cow eats something it should not have like a peice of fencing, it lodges here in the Recticulum. However, the contractions of the reticulum can force the object into the peritoneal cavity where it initiates inflammation. Nails and screws can even peroferate the heart. The grass that has been eaten is also softened further in this stomach section and is formed into small wads of cud. Each cud returns to the cows mouth and is chewed 40 – 60 times and then swallowed properly.

3. The Omasum – this part of the stomach is a 'filter'. It filters through all the food the cow eats. The cud is also pressed and broken down further.

4. The Abomasum – this part of the stomach is like a humans stomach and is connected to the intestines. Here, the food is finally digested by the cows stomach juices and essential nutrients that the cow needs are passed through the bloodstream. The rest is passed through to the intestines and produces a 'cow pat'.

A little poem about the cows stomach!

How Many Udders Does a Cow Have?

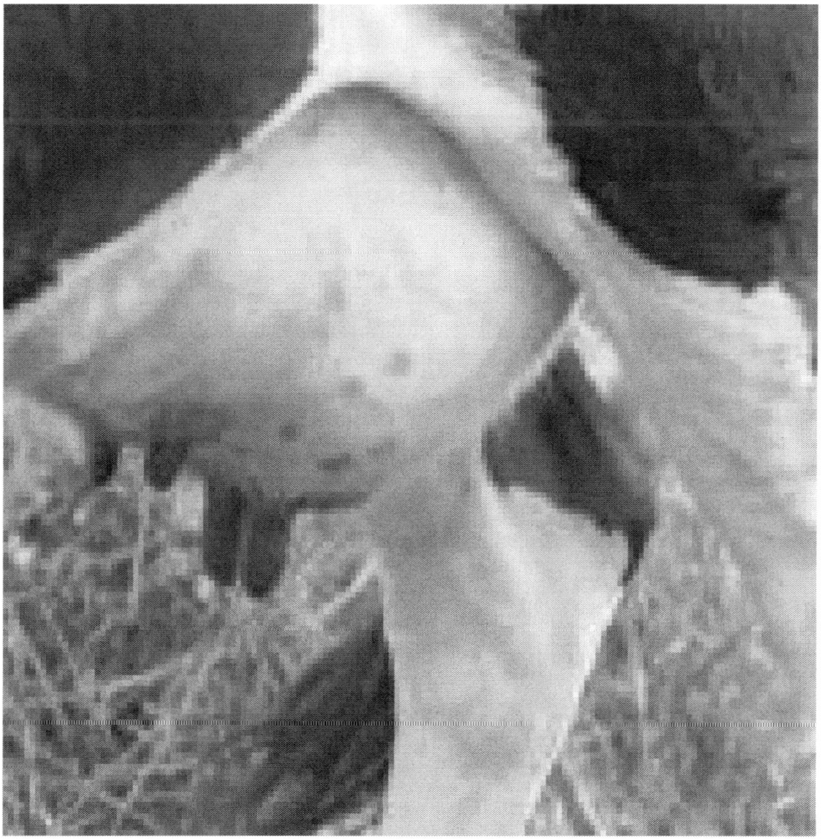

Fig. 1.6

Cows have one udder, which is split into four separate compartments, each containing a separate store of milk. Cows have four teats.

How Many Hearts Does a Cow Have?

Cows have only one heart divided into four sections, just like every other mammal and bird. Cow hearts are bigger than other mammals, so that they can circulate blood around their large bodies

How Many Stomachs Does a Cow Have?

Cows are ruminant animals, they have one stomach with four distinct compartments made up of the Rumen, Reticulum, Omasum and Abomasum

GOAT ANATOMY

Below is an anatomy diagram of a typical female goat.

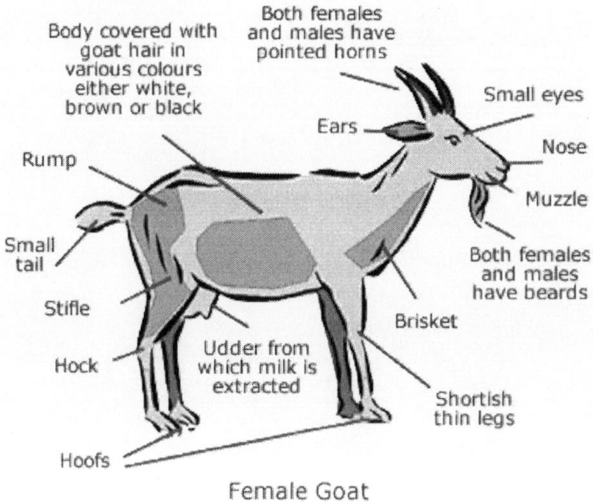

Fig. 1.7

Goats are sure-footed animals who have a rough pad on the bottom of their two-toed hooves. Goats have a long, thick, furry coat that protects them from the cold. Goats range from about 17 to 42 inches (43 to 107 centimetres) tall at the shoulder. Both male and female wild goats have beards and pointed black horns.

Female goats have udders from which goats milk is extracted.

Below is a diagram of the internal digestive system of a goat. It shows the four stomach chambers and the intestines.

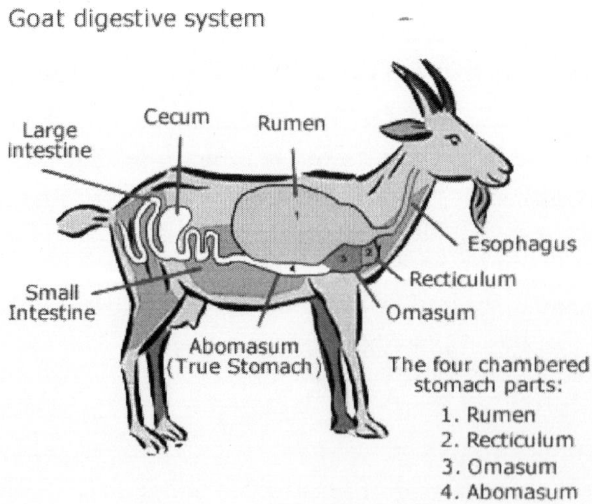

Fig. 1.8

Mature goats are ruminant animals. Their digestive tracts, which are similar to those of cattle, sheep and deer, consist of the mouth, oesophagus, four stomach compartments, small intestine and large intestine.

Like other ruminant animals, goats have no upper incisor or canine teeth. Goats depend on the dental pad in front of the hard palate, lower incisor teeth, lips and tongue to take food into their mouths.

The four chambered stomach explained!

Rumen: This is the largest of the four stomach compartments of ruminant animals. The capacity of the rumen of goats ranges from 3 to 6 gallons depending on the type of feed. This compartment, also known as the 'paunch', contains many microorganisms (bacteria and protozoa) that supply enzymes to breakdown fibre and other food that the goat eats. The conversion of the cellulose of feeds to volatile fatty acids (acetic, propionic, and butyric acids) is the result of microbiological activities in the rumen. These volatile fatty acids are absorbed through the rumen wall and provide up to 80 percent of the total energy requirements of the animal. Microbial digestion in the rumen is the basic reason why ruminant animals effectively utilize fibrous feeds and are maintained primarily on roughages.

Rumen microorganisms also convert components of the feed to useful products such as the essential amino acids, the B complex vitamins, and vitamin K. Finally, the microorganisms themselves are digested further in the digestive tract.

Reticulum: This compartment, also known as the 'hardware stomach' or 'honeycomb', is located just below the entrance of the oesophagus into the stomach. The reticulum is part of the rumen separated only by an overflow connection, the 'rumino-reticular fold'. The capacity of the reticulum of goats ranges from 0.25 to 0.50 gallons.

Omasum: This compartment, also known as the 'manyplies', consists of many folds or layers of tissue that grind up feed ingesta and remove some of the water from the feed. The capacity of the omasum in goats is approximately 0.25 gallons.

Abomasum: This compartment is more often considered the 'true stomach' of ruminant animals. It functions similarly to human stomachs. It contains hydrochloric acid and digestive enzymes that breakdown food particles before they enter the small intestine. The capacity of the abomasum of goats is approximately one gallon.

As partially digested feed enters the small intestine, enzymes produced and secreted by the pancreas and small intestinal mucosa further breakdown feed nutrients into simple compounds that are absorbed into the bloodstream. Undigested feed and unabsorbed nutrients leaving the small intestine pass into the large intestine. The functions of the large intestine include absorption of water and further digestion of feed materials by the microorganisms present in this area. The 100-foot-long intestinal canal of goats has a capacity to hold 3 gallons.

When a goat kid is born, the rumen is small and the abomasum is the largest of the four stomach compartments. The rumen of a goat kid represents about 30 percent of the total stomach area, while the abomasum represents about 70 percent. Hence, digestion in the goat kid is like that of a monogastric animal. In the suckling goat kid, closure of the oesophageal groove ensures that milk is channeled directly to the abomasum, instead of entering the rumen, reticulum, and omasum. When the suckling goat kid starts to eat vegetation (first or second week of life), the rumen, reticulum and omasum gradually develop in size and function.

Goats are very particular about what they eat, they will not consume food of poor quality or food that is dirty or has been trampled on. Goats require the best quality hay, green stuffs and concentrates (oats, barley, soya, linseed, etc. generally sold as a goat mix). However goats will eat a wide range of food, preferring more fibrous food to lush grass. Goats will eat young thistles and brambles, as well as twigs, they also like bark from trees. Goats are inquisitive and will nibble and investigate most items (including the proverbial washing off the line!), however, they are selective about what they actually eat.

HORSE ANATOMY

Horses have, on average, a skeleton of 205 bones. A significant difference in the bones contained in the horse skeleton, as compared to that of a human, is the lack of a collarbone. Their front limb system is attached to the spinal column by a powerful set of muscles, tendons and ligaments that attach the shoulder blade to the torso.

The horses legs and hooves are also unique, interesting structures. Their leg bones are proportioned differently from those of a human. For example, the body part that is called a horses 'knee' is actually the carpal bones that correspond to the human wrist. Similarly, the hock contains the bones equivalent to those in the human ankle and heel.

The lower leg bones of a horse correspond to the bones of the human hand or foot. The fetlock (incorrectly called the 'ankle') is actually the proximal sesamoid bones (bones that are typically found in locations where a tendon passes over a joint) between the cannon bones (a single equivalent to the human metacarpal (the intermediate part of the hand skeleton) or metatarsal bones (five long bones of the foot)) and the proximal phalanges (bones found in the limbs of most vertebrates), located where one finds the 'knuckles' of a human. A horse also has no muscles in its legs below the knees and hocks, only skin and hair, bone, tendons, ligaments, cartilage and the assorted specialized tissues that make up the hoof.

The skeleton gives support for the muscles, protection for the internal organs, and possesses the necessary mobility of its parts for the horse to move at various speeds or lie down or graze.

Below is a diagram of the some of the most important bones within a horse:

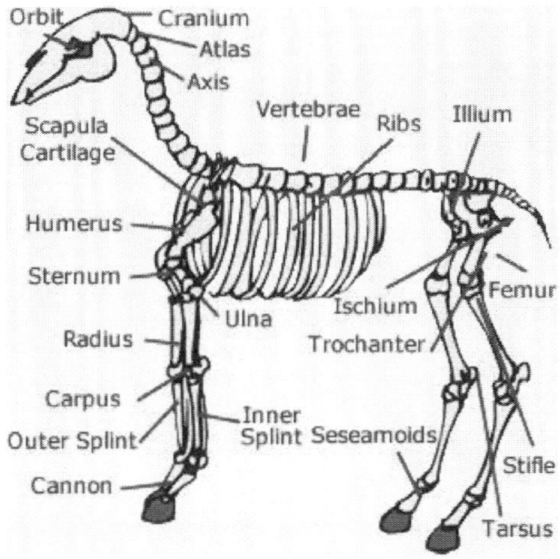

Fig. 1.9

Below is a diagram of a horses body parts – the numbers on the diagram correspond with the body part names:

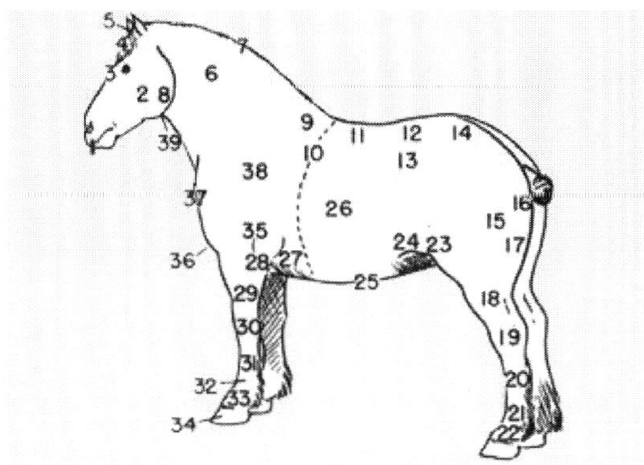

Fig. 1.10

1. muzzle 2. cheek 3. face 4. forehead 5. poll 6. neck 7. crest 8.jaw 9. withers 10. heart girth 11. back 12. loin 13. coupling 14. croup 15. thigh 16. point of buttock 17. quarters 18. gaskin 19. hock 20. cannon 21. fetlock joint 22. pastern 23. stifle 24. rear flank 25. under line 26. ribs 27. fore flank 28. elbow 29. forearm 30. knee 31. cannon 32. fetlock joint 33. pastern 34. foot 35. arm 36. breast 37. point of shoulder 38. shoulder 39. throat latch

ELEPHANT ANATOMY

The elephants body is well adapted for the survival of rugged conditions of their habitats in Africa and Asia. Elephants have strong, long trunks that perform multiple tasks, sharp tusks used for carrying heavy objects and for fighting with, large ears which they flap to keep themselves cool as well as having other functions. Elephants also have a tail that with one swish can whisk away flies and other insects making it the perfect fly swatter.

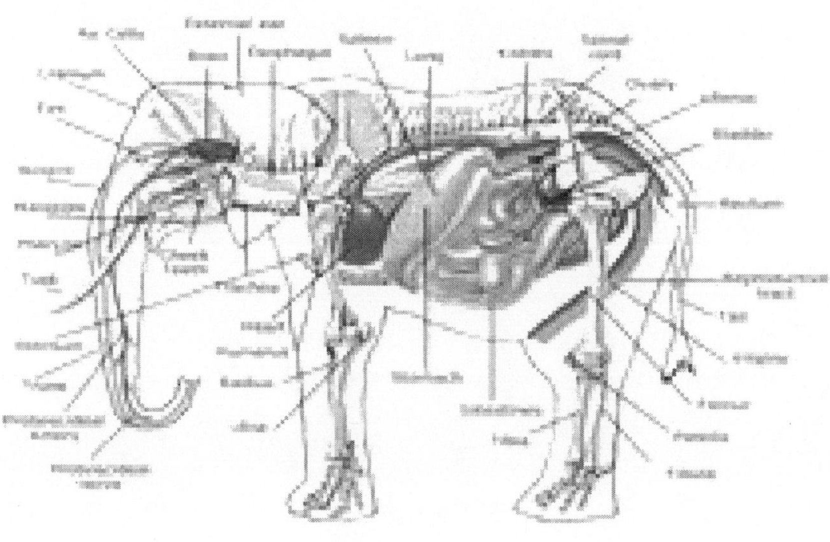

Fig. 1.11

On the left is an anatomy diagram of the internal organs of a female elephant. Click on the image for a larger look at it.

The larger image will open in a new window, use the close button when finished.

Below you can see some distinct differences between the African elephant and the Asian elephants body structures. The African is larger, with much larger ears and larger all round in height and length. For more detailed information on either the African Elephant or the Asian Elephant, click on the individual images in the picture below.

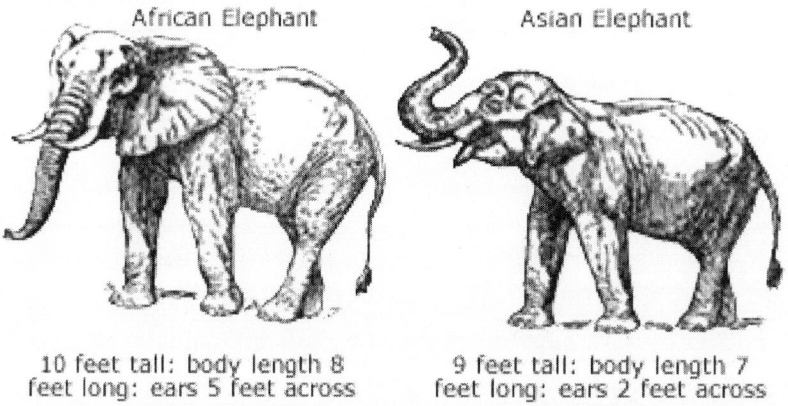

Fig. 1.12

Elephant Trunks

One of the most interesting features of an elephant is its trunk. An elephants trunk is both an upper lip and an extension of the nose with two nostrils running through the whole length.

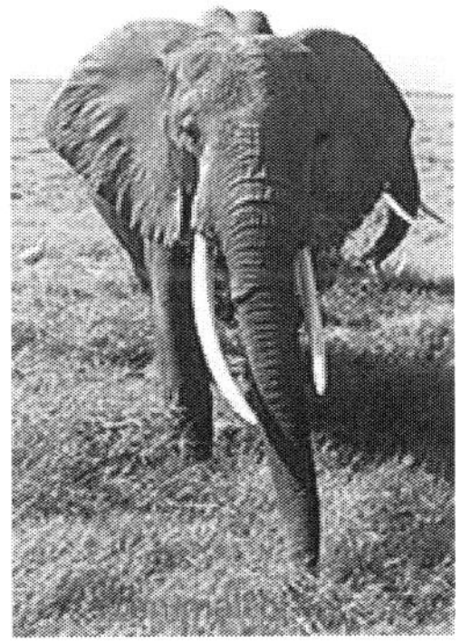

Fig. 1.13

The trunk has more than 40,000 muscles in it which is more than a human has in their whole body. A human being only has 639 muscles in total. An elephants trunk is both strong and very agile. It can perform multiple tasks from pushing over heavy trees to picking up the smallest twig. An elephant uses its trunk to pick up and throw objects, rub an itchy eye or ear, fills it with water and then pours it into its mouth to drink and also as a snorkel when swimming under water. Elephants also use it for feeding and for friendly wrestling matches with other elephants.

The trunk plays an important role in an elephants life by being used as an exploratory organ. The trunk is extremely flexible and can be used with the finest touch. At the first sign of danger, an elephant raises its trunk to smell the air and detect the smell of what is threatening. An elephant uses a whole range of smelling tasks as it is one of the elephants primary sensory organs, along with the ears. An elephants trunk is so important and vital to its life that it would be almost impossible for the elephant to survive should it ever get damaged.

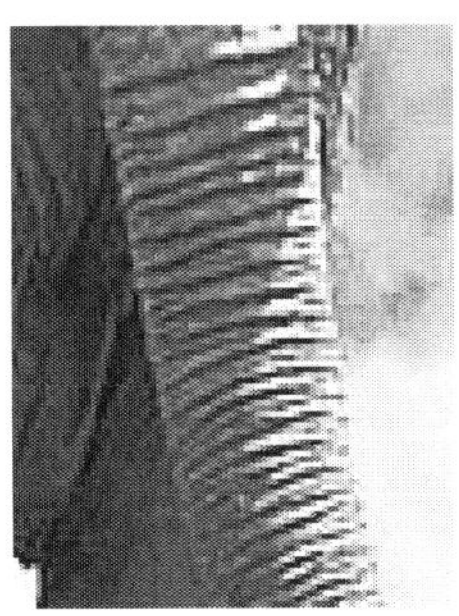

Fig. 1.14

Most animals use their nose solely for breathing, however, the elephant also uses its trunk for water storage and for drawing in mud and dust to spray over themselves to clean or cool down. An average elephant can hold and store 4 litres of water inside its trunk. The trunk has a sparse covering of fine sensory hairs and the skin covering the front of the trunk has rings of deep crevasses and resembles a slinky.

The African elephant has two prehensile fingers at the tip of its trunk which are used to grab hold of objects and smaller items. The Asian elephant has only one finger at the end of its trunk and usually only uses its trunk to scoop things up. Elephants can lift very heavy weights with its trunk, but it is important to remember that each elephant is individual and unique and the amount of weight each can lift varies. The trunk is not usually used in combat or for fighting with, but it can be used to make threatening gestures. However, elephants do use their trunks to play fight which can be quite interesting to observe.

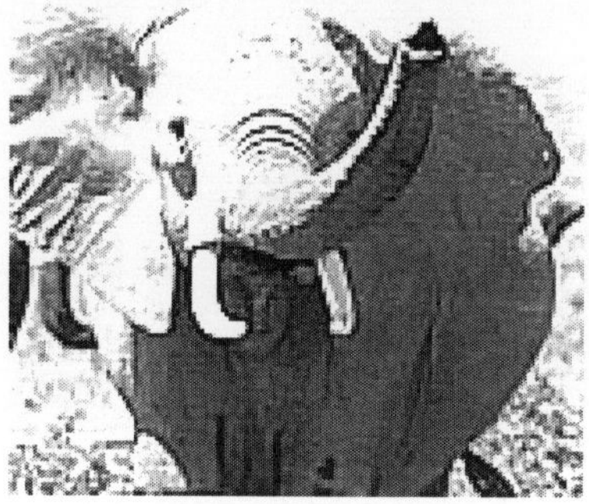

Fig. 1.15

Another interesting observation is when an elephant is charging. If its trunk is stretched out in front, then the elephant is just bluffing. However, it the trunk is curled or tucked downwards then it means business and is serious about its intentions. Like all vertebrates, elephants possess the Jacobson's organ in its mouth (a smelling organ).

The elephant tests and experiments with different odours by touching a particular object with its trunk and then placing the trunk in its mouth. Elephants are very inquisitive creatures.

Elephant tusks are very elongated incisor teeth. Elephants do not have any canine teeth at all. Both male and female African elephants have tusks, however, only the male species of the Asian elephant has them. Tusks continue growing for most of the elephants life. They are an age indicator – much like the elephants feet, the age of the elephant can be estimated by observing their tusks. The size of an elephants tusks is an inherited characteristic, however, because of ivory hunters, it would be quite rare today to find and elephant whose tusks weigh more than 100 pounds.

The total length of the tusks is not apparent on the outside of the elephant, about a third of the length of the tusk lies hidden inside the elephants skull. This is the unfortunate reason ivory hunters destroy the elephant for their tusks instead of just cutting them off. Ivory is really only dentine and is no different from ordinary teeth. It is the diamond shaped pattern of the elephants tusk which can be distinguished when viewed from a cross-section which gives elephant ivory its distinctive lustre.

Elephants are either 'left-tusked' or 'right-tusked', just like a human being might be 'left-handed' or 'right-handed'. The favoured tusk is usually shorter than the other due to constant use. Tusks on an individual elephant can differ in shape, length, thickness and growth direction. Male elephants tend to have heavier, longer and more stouter tusks than females do.

An elephant uses its tusks to many many tasks just like its trunk. They use their tusks for digging, ripping bark of trees, foraging, carrying heavy objects and for resting a wary, heavy trunk on. They will also use them as weapons should they ever encounter conflict.

Tusks in a baby elephant (Calf) are present at birth and are really only like milk teeth. They measure only about 5 centimetres long. These 'milk tusks' will fall out around their first birthday. Their permanent tusks will then start to protrude beyond their lips at around 2 – 3 years old and will continue to grow throughout their lives.

Tusks grow at about 15 – 18 centimetres per year, however, they are continually worn down with constant use. Should they be allowed to continually grow without use, they would grow into a spiral shape (similar to those of the extinct woolly mammoth) as they typically grow following a curved growth pattern.

Interestingly, some elephants are born without tusks. This hereditary condition causes huge differences in the musculature and shape of the neck and the head of the elephant. Also, the carriage of the head is different and the bones at the back of the skull are less developed.

Not all male Asian elephants have tusks, there is approximately 40 – 50% of male Asian elephants that are tuskless. These particular males are known as 'Makhnas' in India.

Elephant Teeth

An elephants teeth are very unique in the manner in which they proceed from the back of each half jaw towards the front. The teeth follow a linear progression. As the front teeth continuously become more worn down they are slowly replaced with new teeth that give the elephant an ability to chew the coarse foods it eats particularly tree bark. The elephant has a total of 24 teeth, but only 2 are usually in use at any one time.

When an elephant is born, a calf has four developing teeth in each side of its jaws. These consist of their smallish first and second teeth which are present after birth and the end of a third and a forth which is still below the gum. As each tooth wears out, it is pushed forward to the front of the mouth and it slowly wears into a shelf as the roots are absorbed. The shelf eventually will break off and the remaining piece will be pushed out of the mouth.

After the first two teeth are gone, parts of the two adjacent teeth are being worn down in each half of the jaw. This process continues until the 6th and sometimes 7th molar appears. The 6th molar weighs on average an incredible 4 kilograms and has a maximum grinding length of 21 centimetres (and a width of 7 centimetres). This 6th molar will be present for around half the elephants life. When the last molar tooth is worn down and the elephant can no longer chew properly, unfortunately it will usually starve or develop malnutrition and eventually die. This does not happen until the elephant is at least 60 – 70 years old. Below is a table showing the onset and loss of each tooth and age the above process usually occurs:

Molar Molar Appearance Molar Loss 1 At birth 2 years old 2 At birth 6 years old 3 1 year old 13 – 15 years old 4 6 years old 28 years old 5 18 years old 43 years old 6 30 years old 65 years old +

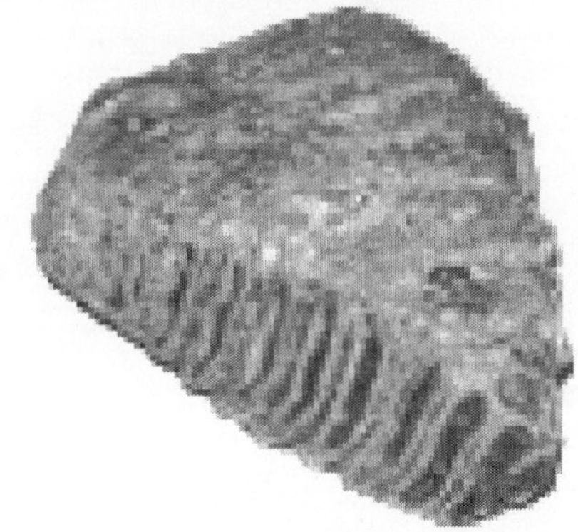

Fig. 1.16

The molars of an elephant differ between the African and Asian species. Both have a series of ridges (laminae) which run across the tooth. However, in the Asian elephant the ridges are parallel as opposed to the diamond shaped ridges in the African elephant. Although the Asian elephant has grazing teeth, it is usually spends most of its time in forests as opposed to plains like the African elephant.

In both species of elephant, the movement of the jaw during chewing is forwards and backwards, unlike cows who use sideways movements to chew their cud. Therefore, the ridges act as two rasps grating upon one another and is made more effective by the teeth being slightly curved along the lengths.

Elephants Brain

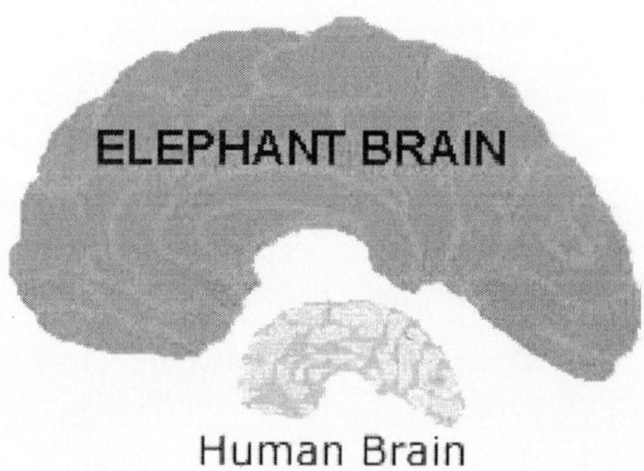

Fig. 1.17

The brain of the elephant is larger than any other land mammal and is located in the back of the skull well away from the forehead. An elephants brain is about four times the size of a humans brain. (See diagram on the left). Out of all the animals that have ever lived on earth, the brain of the elephant is the largest known.

Elephants are born with 35% of the mass of the adult brain. The elephant is among the more intelligent animals. The brain weight of the male African elephant is 4.2-5.4 kilograms. The brain weight of the female African elephant is 3.6 – 4.3 kilograms. Both are quite heavy in comparison to the adult human brain although brain development in elephants is quite similar to that of human beings.

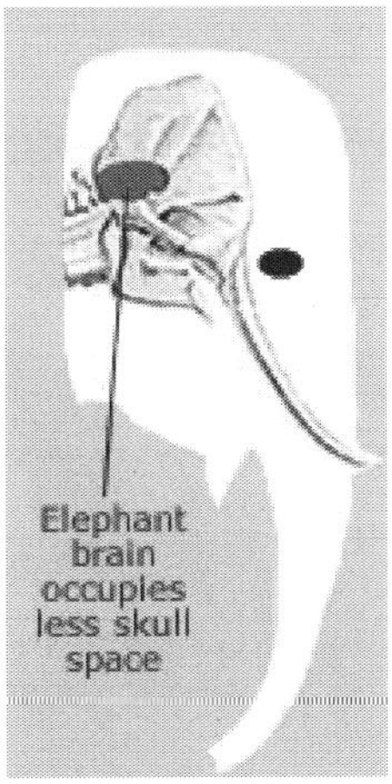

Fig. 1.18

Humans are born with small brain mass, so are elephants. As a human brain grows and develops, so does an elephant calfs brain. Likewise, the learning ability of a human increases with growth, so does that of an elephant calf. It is not surprising that elephants are such intelligent creatures. Although the female elephant brain is smaller than the male elephant brain, this does not suggest that the male is more intelligent than the female. Studies have revealed that the female elephant is equal to or even more intelligent than the male. Given the fact that female elephants are generally smaller to male elephants, the brain mass in proportion to the body size indicates the larger female brain.

Also, the brain and consciousness of the female elephant is much different than that of a male as they are reared and interact with their mothers in very different ways right from birth and while the females form a very close knit bond with each other which is constantly maintained, the males are more solitary and independent.

Although the brain of the elephant is the largest in size among all of the land mammals, it actually only occupies a small area at the back of the skull. However, in proportion to the size of the elephants body, the elephant brain is smaller than the human brain. Despite this, the elephant is one of the only animals along with all apes (including ourselves), sperm whales and a few other creatures who has a large brain relative to body size.

Elephant Hair

Although elephants are generally considered hairless animals, both African and Asian elephants are born with thick hair. The elephant fetus is covered with 'Lanugo', a mass of long, downy hair, however, most of this is shed before the elephant is actually born. The hair on an elephant calf sheds more as the elephant calf grows. The hair is not designed to provide warmth for the elephant, however, it does allow the elephant to sense the closeness of objects the hair touches.

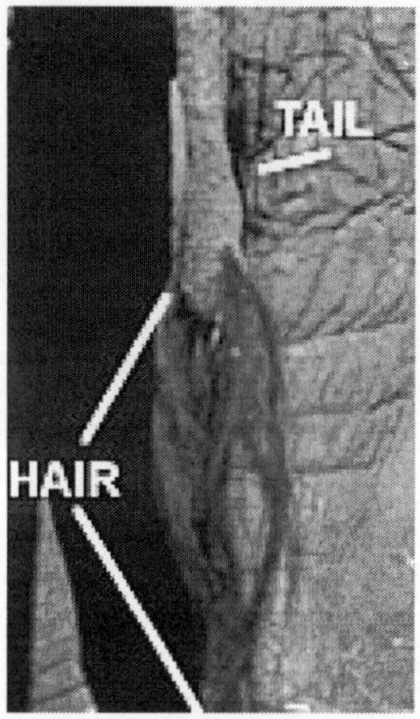

Fig. 1.19

The hair on an elephant is thickest on the tail and more visible on the head and back. The hair on the tail can reach a length of up to 100 centimetres.

The hair that appears around the eyes and nose have a protection purpose. It helps to keep out particles and germs from invading the body through the ears and nose. An elephant also has small sensory hairs along its trunk.

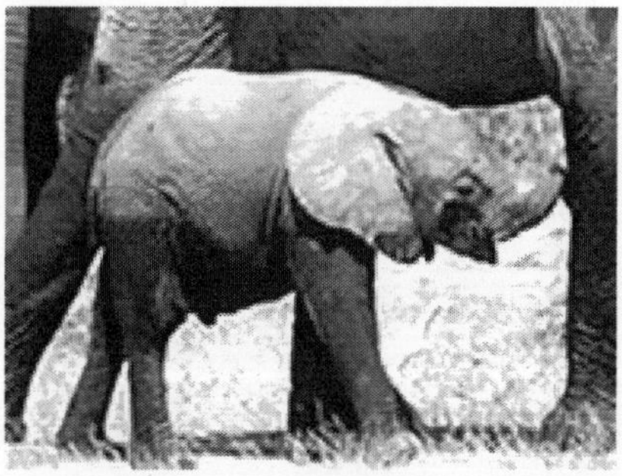

Fig.1.20

Baby elephants (calves) have lots of small fine hairs that cover most of their body. In the photo on the left, you can see the fine hair on the calfs forehead and lower back. These hairs will last in the same density long after the elephants first birthday and then as the elephant grows the hair will gradually become thinner and become less visible.

Elephant Ears

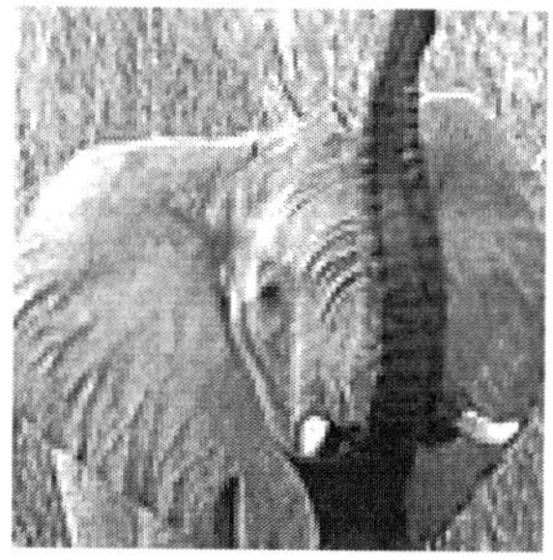

Fig.1.21

The African elephant has ears that are at least 3 times the size of the Asian elephants ears. The African elephant uses its ears as signaling organs. Ears are also used to regulate body temperature and are used as a protective feature in the African elephant to ward off potential threats. Each elephants ear is unique and different to any other elephants ear. They are used just like fingerprints on a human as a type of identification. The ears serve several important functions in the elephant. When a threat is perceived by the elephant, the ears are spread wide on each side of the head, which produces a huge frontal area.

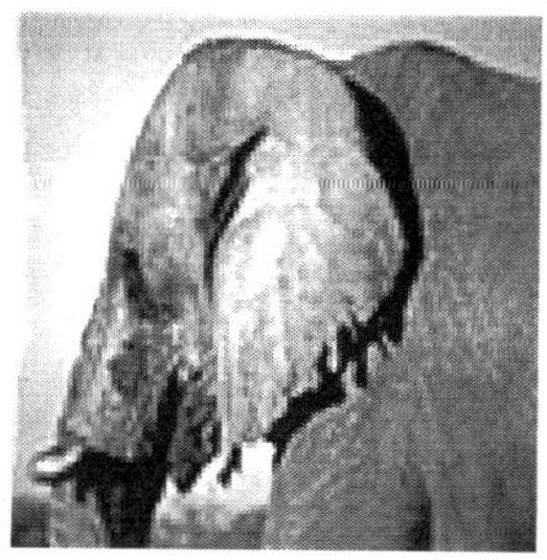

Fig. 1.22 a

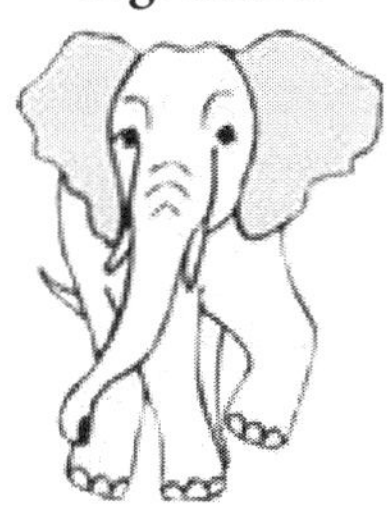

Fig. 1.22 b

Because the elephant is such a large bulbous shape and contains large organs, their insides generate a lot of heat, particularly the digestive system. The surface area of an elephant is a lower ratio compared to the elephants volume. Therefore, there is not enough skin area to cope with the heat that needs expelling. So elephants use their ears to perform this function. When an elephant flaps its ears, it can lower their blood temperature by 10 degrees Fahrenheit . Both the African and Asian elephants use their ears for this purpose although it is more effective in the African elephant due to the larger ears.

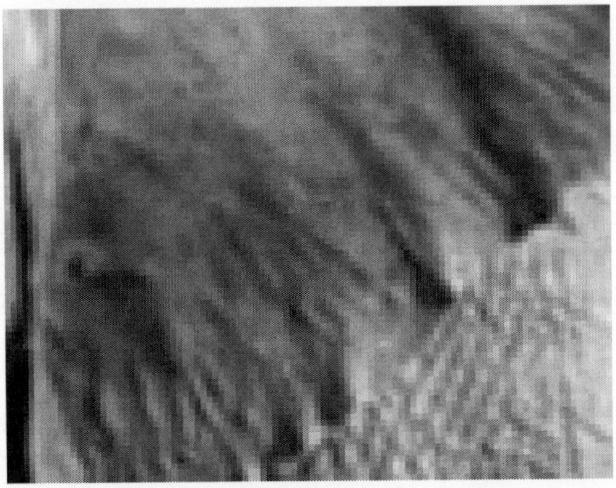

Fig. 1.23

The wider surface area of outer ear tissue on the African elephants ears consists of a vast network of capillaries and veins. Hot blood in the arteries are filtered through these and cooler blood is returned to the elephants body.

It is not uncommon to see an elephant facing down on a windy day with its ears extended to allow the cool wind to blow across the hot arteries. The physical structure of the elephant ear is simply a sheet of cartilage covered by thin skin. Another amazing function of the elephant ear is its 'infra sound capabilities'. This is used for long range communication between the elephants. Elephant ears are extremely sensitive and studies have proved that elephants can communicate over great distances with each other. Elephants can use this communication which is unhearing to human ears to warn of impending dangers in the far distance. So do not forget, if you have the opportunity to ever touch the ears of an elephant, be very careful as they are very soft and sensitive.

Elephant Feet

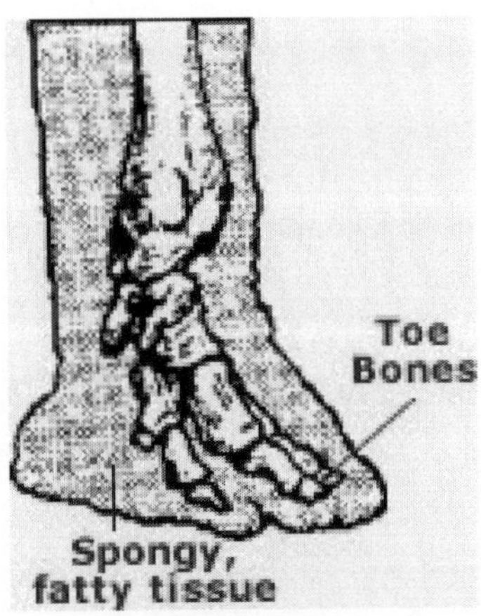

Fig. 1.24

Elephants feet are unique and very interesting. They are quite different from other animal feet. An elephants foot is designed in such a way that elephants actually walk on the tips of their toes. Because of the way it walks, elephants are also known as 'Digitigrades' and belong to a group of animals that also includes horses, cattle, sheep, camels and rhinos. All elephants do not have the same number of toes on each foot. The African elephants have 4 toes on their front feet and 3 toes on their back feet. Asian elephants on the other hand, have 5 on the front and 4 at the back.

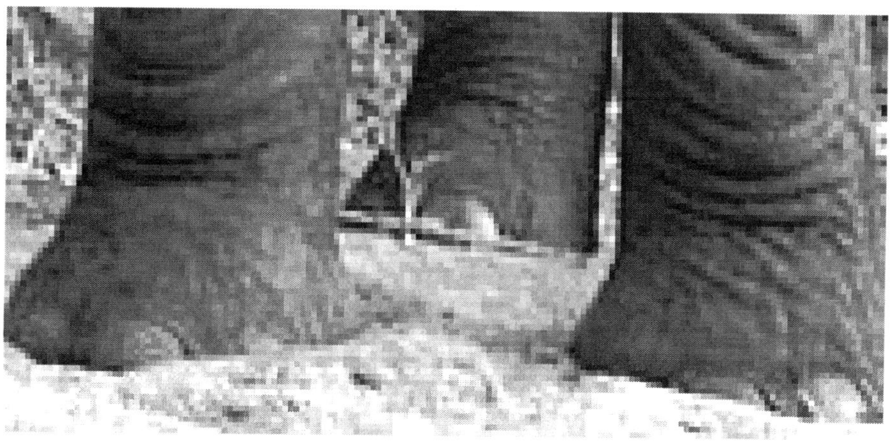

Fig. 1.25

Elephants toes are buried inside of the flesh of the foot and not all toes have toenails. An elephants foot generally measures 40 – 50 centimetres in length and width and has a circumference of about 1.34 metres. The sole of an elephants foot is made of a tough, fatty connective tissue which acts like a spongy shock absorber and allows the elephant to move about silently.

The sole of the foot is also ridged and pitted which gives the elephant stability when walking over a variety of terrains. Its design prevents the elephant from slipping on smooth surfaces such as ice and snow. The reason that elephants can walk so quietly is in part due to the 'elastic spongy cushion' on the bottom of the foot smothering any objects beneath itself. This causes most noises (including the cracking of sticks and twigs) to be muffled.

The fore feet of an elephant have a circular shape whereas the back feet are a more oval shape. The footprint of an elephant can tell you a few things about that particular elephant. For example, elongated oval footprints usually indicates that they belong to a male elephant, whereas a more rounded footprint indicates a female elephant. Male elephants tend to leave double footprints as their rear leg falls slightly to the side of their front leg. Females tend to walk more precisely in the same spot with both legs.

The footprint can also tell you what age the elephant might be. Younger elephants leave a more crisp and defined footprint. Older elephants leave a more undefined footprint because of smoother ridges and worn heels. The height of the elephant can also be determined by its footprint. Twice the circumference of the footprint suggests how tall the elephant is to the height of its shoulder. Elephants footprints can play a beneficial role for other animals. Their large, deep prints create holes in which water can be collected in providing water holes for small animals, roots can be dug up from the ground and navigation on difficult terrain can be made easier.

The structure of the foot allows an elephant to walk in deep mud without difficulty, because when it is being withdrawn the circumference becomes smaller which in turn reduces the suction preventing the elephant from being drawn deeper into the mud.

Lephant Skin

Although elephants belong to the Pachyderm species which means 'thick-skinned' animals, they actually have very thin skin except in certain places such as the back and the sides where it is about 2 – 3 centimetres thick. The thinnest parts of skin are behind their ears, around their eyes, on the chest, abdomen and shoulders. On these parts, their skin is as thin as paper. Skin provides a protective function for all animals, however, there are some unique characteristics about the elephants skin. Elephants skin is very sensitive to the sun. Elephant calves are constantly shadowed by their mothers to avoid sunburn.

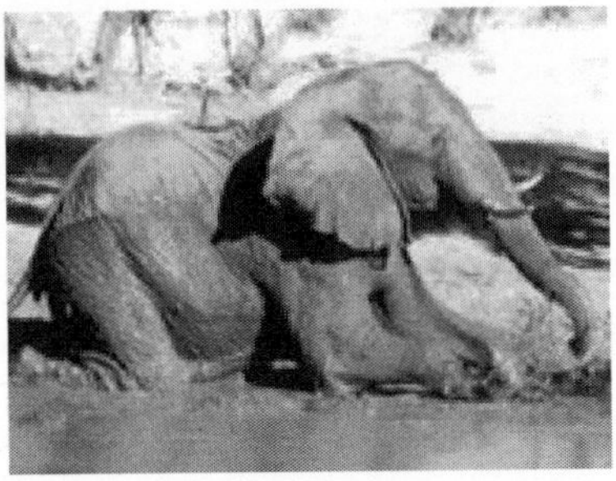

Fig. 1.26

Elephants naturally love water, however, one of the reasons they enjoy wallowing in mud, lakes and rivers is to keep cool when it is very hot. Elephants also use their trunks to draw up cool water and squirt it over their backs and heads to wet the skin most exposed to the sunlight. The absence of sweat glands is also another important reason for elephants to spend a lot of time in water and mud.

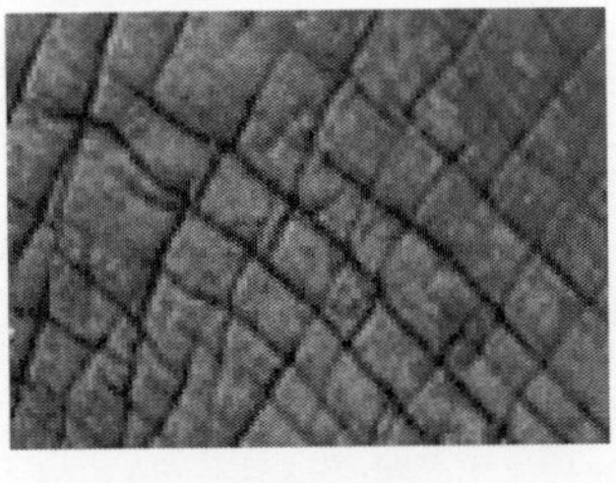

Fig. 1.27

An elephants skin is so sensitive and rich in nerves that it can detect even the smallest fly landing upon it. As we all know, elephants skin is very wrinkly. These wrinkles have their purpose too. They help the elephant in controlling its body temperature and keeping itself cool.

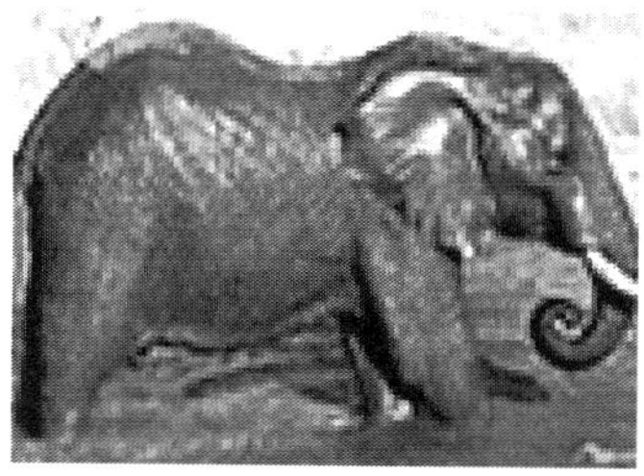

Fig. 1.28

Wrinkles increase the surface area of the skin so when the elephant bathes in water, there is more skin to wet. When the elephant comes out of the water, the cracks and crevices of the wrinkles trap the water and because it takes longer to evaporate in the heat it keeps the elephants skin moist longer than it would if it had smooth skin.

Skin structure on an elephant can also distinguish whether they are Asian or African. Asian elephants have finer skin than African elephants and it is sometimes colorless except for some 'white spots' around the ears and forehead.

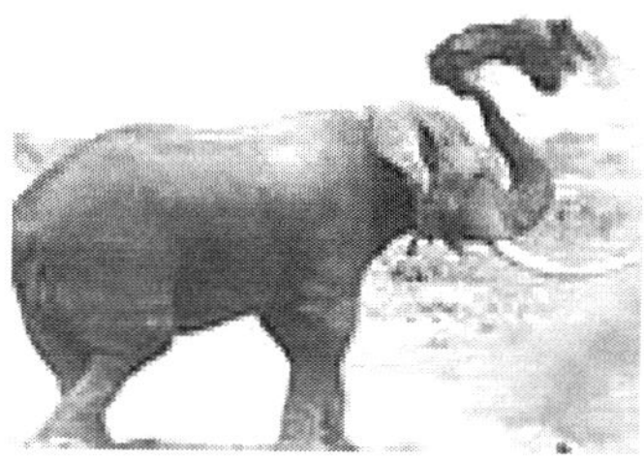

Fig. 1.29

The natural skin color of the African elephant is greyish black, but all elephant skin color changes and is determined by the color of the soil of the land where their habitat is. Elephants have a habit of throwing mud over their backs and this gives them their apparent coloring.

Elephant Senses and Communication

By better understanding an elephants view of the world we can become more aware of how amazing these animals really are. As human beings, the impact our senses have on the nature of our experiences such as what we see, hear, smell and touch, play a huge part in determining our world. Likewise, it is important that we recognize the world of an elephant is much different from our world. For instance, the eyesight of an elephant is not as far reaching as a humans eyesight, however, an elephants sense of smell is unparalleled.

The elephants acute sense of smell is also used in communication along with its other senses of vision, touch, hearing and the amazing ability to detect vibrations.

An elephant is capable of hearing sound waves well below the human hearing limitation. They communicate using both high and low frequency sounds. Low frequency rumbles are made to warn other elephants at long distance of a current situation whereas high frequency sounds such as trumpeting, barking, snorting and other loud calls are used to communicate to those nearer.

Using their heads, bodies, trunks, ears and tail for communicating is the elephants natural language. Visual communication includes movements of the head, mouth, tusks and trunk. For example, when a female elephant feels threatened, she will make herself appear larger by holding her head as high as she can and spreading her ears wide. Chemical communication is the use of the trunk. The elephant will lift its trunk to smell the air or root around the floor usually searching for urine spots and urine trails.

Tactile communication usually involves the whole body, feet, tail, ears, trunk and tusks and is mostly to do with touch. An elephant will use its tusks to provoke aggression or to lift a baby elephant out of a mud wallow. The rubbing together of ears shows affection. Depending on how the elephant moves and uses its body parts depicts the mood of the animal. Such moods and body movements show if the elephant is angry, happy, anti-predator, parental, excited or sad. Every observation of the elephant senses shows an insight to the world the elephant lives in. It is important to remember that the elephants world is a completely different world from ours based on its sensory experiences.

2

BIRD ANATOMY

All birds have the same basic skeletal structure but with different variations in size and shape depending upon species. A bird skeleton is very unique whether the bird is flightless or adapted for flight. The skeletal structure is very lightweight and can appear fragile, however, it is actually very strong and robust. Most of the longer bones of the bird's skeleton are hollow but reinforced through a honeycombed substructure of criss-crossing for structural strength.

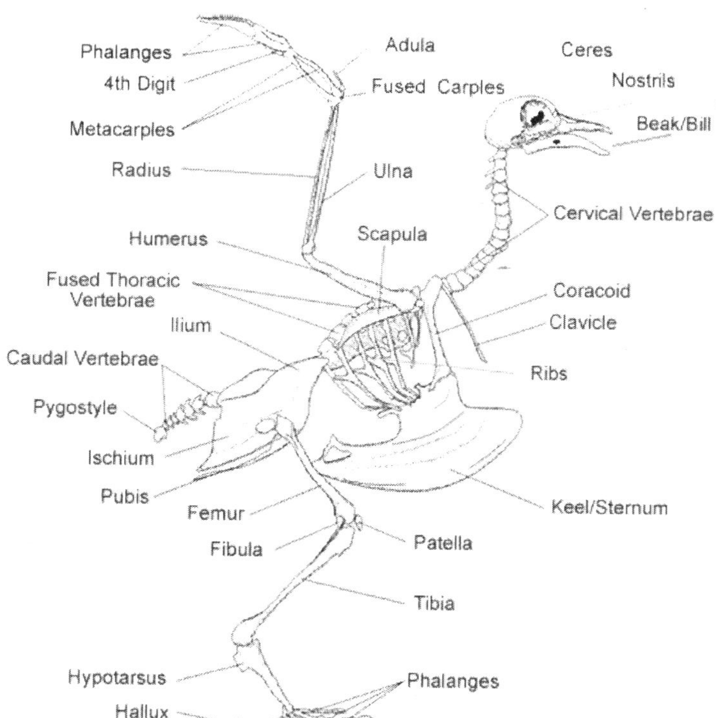

Fig 2.1

When birds flap their wings, it requires much strength from large muscles which need to be solidly attached to the skeleton. Flying birds have a pronounced keel or sternum, the flight muscles are attached to this. Fused bones also helps the bird to withstand the stress of taking off, flying and landing. The keel is absent in flightless birds such as Penguins, Emus and Ostriches who also have solid bones instead of hollow ones.

The leg bones of birds are the heaviest, contributing to a low centre of gravity. This gives the bird a better balance, important in both flight and bipedal (two legged) locomotion. A bird's skeleton comprises only about 5% of its total body weight.

The Internal Anatomy of a Bird

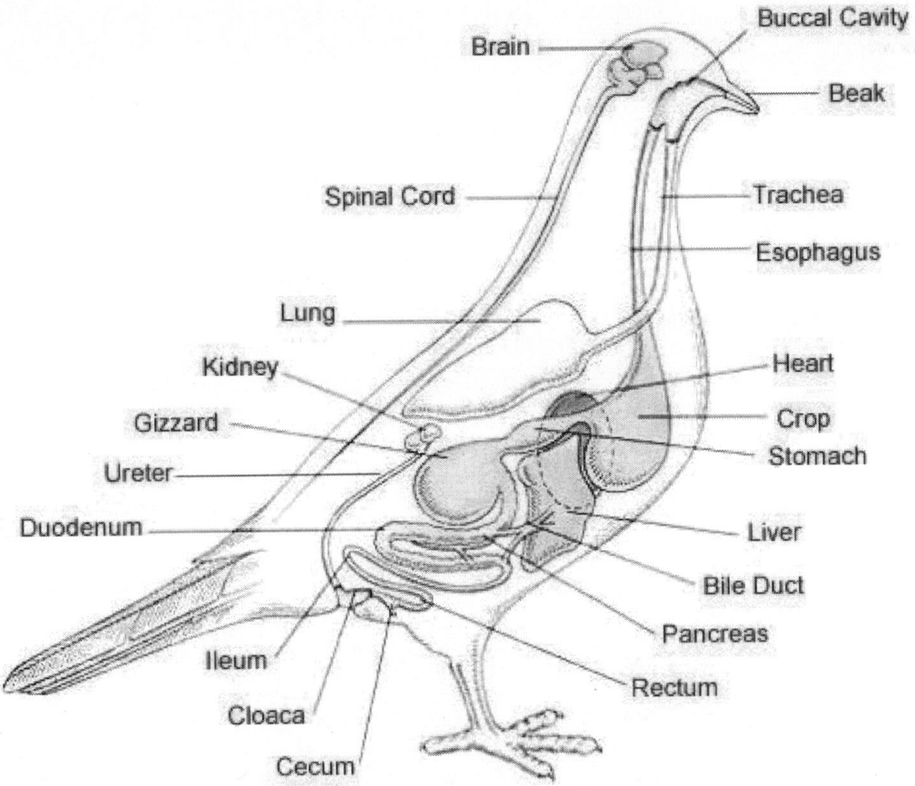

Fig. 2.2

Bird Respiratory System

A bird's internal anatomy, particularly its respiratory system, differs from mammals in many ways. Bird respiration is much more efficient.

- Birds do not have a diaphram like mammals which mammals use to increase and decrease their chest cavity. Instead, birds push their sternum in and out which produces the same effect.

- Breathing rate varies depending on the size of the bird. For example, a hummingbird breathes 143 times per minute while a turkey breathes 7 times per minute. This rate increases when birds are flying. The flow of air enters through the nostrils, down the trachea and into the lungs and air sacs.
- The lungs of birds are very compact and occupy much less space than the lungs of mammals. With the help of thin-walled air sacs which extend through the body cavity and even into the bones, birds can keep a continuous flow of air through the lungs.

Digestive System

Because birds have a beak or bill and no teeth, they do not really chew their food and therefore have a specialised digestive tract.

- When a bird eats, the food firstly travels down the esophagus and into the crop which is really just an extension of the esophagus. The food is held in the crop before it can enter the proventriculus which produces acids and enzymes to help break down the food. The food then passes into the gizzard which breaks down tough foods such as seeds and nuts.
- Did you know that the Turkey has one of the most remarkable gizzards which can breakdown the most toughest foods such as walnuts. It can even breakdown objects that the Turkey may have eaten such as steel needles and other metal objects.
- A bird's gizzard contains keratin to make the surface rough. Keratin is a substance which makes up human hair and fingernails and is what Rhino's horns are made off.
- When the bird's food has been ground up in the gizzard, it travels through the intestines where nutrients are absorbed. Waste is then expelled through the cloaca.

Chemicals

The elements (simplest chemical substances) found in an animal's body are all made of basic building blocks or atoms. The most common elements found in cells are given in the table below with the symbol that is used to represent them.

Atom	Symbol
Calcium	Ca
Carbon	C
Chlorine	Cl
Copper	Cu
Iodine	I

Hydrogen	H
Iron	Fe
Magnesium	Mg
Nitrogen	N
Atom	Symbol
Oxygen	O
Phosphorous	P
Potassium	K
Sodium	Na
Sulfur	S
Zinc	Zn

Compounds And Molecules

A compound or molecule is formed when two or more atoms join together. Note that some atoms are never found alone. For example oxygen is always found as molecules of 2 oxygen atoms (represented as $O2$).

The table below gives some common compounds.

Compound	Symbol
Calcium carbonate	$CaCO3$
Carbon dioxide	$CO2$
Copper sulfate	$CuSO4$
Glucose	$C6H12O6$
Hydrochloric acid	HCl
Sodium bicarbonate (baking soda)	$NaHCO3$
Sodium chloride (table salt)	NaCl
Sodium hydroxide	NaOH
Water	$H2O$

Chemical Reactions

Reactions occur when atoms combine with or separate from other atoms. In the process new products with different chemical properties are formed.

Chemical reactions can be represented by chemical equations. The starting atoms or compounds are usually put on the left-hand side of the equation and the products on the right-hand side.

For example

- $H2O + CO2$ gives $H2CO3$

- Water + Carbon dioxide gives Carbonic acid

Ionization

When some atoms dissolve in water they become charged particles called ions. Some become positively charged ions and others negatively charged. Ions may have one, two or sometimes three charges.

The table below shows examples of positively and negatively charged ions with the number of their charges.

Positive Ions	Negative Ions		
H+	Hydrogen	Cl-	Chloride
Ca+	Calcium	OH-	Hydroxyl
Na+	Sodium	HCO3-	Bicarbonate
K+	Potassium	CO3-	Carbonate
Mg+	Magnesium	SO4-	Sulfate
Fe+	Iron (ferrous)	PO4-	Phosphate
Fe+	Iron (ferric)	S-	Sulfide

Positive and negative ions attract one another to hold compounds together.

Ions are important in cells because they conduct electricity when dissolved in water. Substances that ionise in this way are known as electrolytes.

The molecules in an animal's body fall into two groups: inorganic compounds and organic compounds. The difference between these is that the first type does not contain carbon and the second type does.

Organic And Inorganic Compounds

Inorganic compounds include water, sodium chloride, potassium hydroxide and calcium phosphate.

Water is the most abundant inorganic compound, making up over 60% of the volume of cells and over 90% of body fluids like blood. Many substances dissolve in water and all the chemical reactions that take place in the body do so when dissolved in water. Other inorganic molecules help keep the acid/base balance (pH) and concentration of the blood and other body fluids stable (8).

Organic compounds include carbohydrates, proteins and fats. All organic molecules contain carbon atoms and they tend to be larger and more complex molecules than inorganic ones. This is largely because each carbon atom can link with four other atoms. Organic compounds can therefore consist of from one to many thousands of carbon atoms joined to form chains, branched chains and rings. All organic compounds also contain hydrogen and they may also contain other elements.

Carbohydrates

The name "carbohydrate" tells you something about the composition of these "hydrated carbon" compounds. They contain carbon, hydrogen and oxygen and like water (H2O), there are always twice as many hydrogen atoms as oxygen atoms in each molecule. Carbohydrates are a large and diverse group that includes sugars, starches, glycogen and cellulose. Carbohydrates in the diet supply an animal with much of its energy and in the animal's body, they transport and store energy.

Carbohydrates are divided into three major groups based on size: monosaccharides (single sugars), disaccharides (double sugars) and polysaccharides (multi sugars).

Monosaccharides are the smallest carbohydrate molecules. The most important monosaccharide is glucose which supplies much of the energy in the cell. It consists of a ring of 6 carbon atoms with oxygen and hydrogen atoms attached.

Disaccharides are formed when 2 monosaccharides join together. Sucrose (table sugar), maltose, and lactose (milk sugar), are three important disaccharides. They are broken down to monosaccharides by digestive enzymes in the gut.

Polysaccharides like starch, glycogen and cellulose are formed by tens or hundreds of monosaccharides linking together. Unlike mono- and di-saccharides, polysaccharides are not sweet to taste and most do not dissolve in water.

Disaccharide (Lactose)

- Starch is the main molecule in which plants store the energy gained from the sun. It is found in grains like barley and roots like potatoes.
- Glycogen, the polysaccharide used by animals to store energy, is found in the liver and the muscles that move the skeleton.
- Cellulose forms the rigid cell walls of plants. Its structure is similar to glycogen, but it can't be digested by mammals. Cows and horses can eat cellulose with the help of bacteria which live in specialised parts of their gut.

Fats

Fats or lipids are important in the plasma membrane around cells and form the insulating fat layer under the skin. They are also a highly concentrated source of energy, and when eaten in the diet provide twice as much energy per gram as either carbohydrates or proteins.

Like carbohydrates fats contain carbon, hydrogen and oxygen, but unlike them, there is no particular relationship between the number of hydrogen and oxygen atoms.

The fats and oils animals eat in their diets are called triglycerides or neutral fats. The building blocks of triglycerides are 3 fatty acids attached to a backbone of glycerol (glycerine). When fats are eaten the digestive enzymes break down the molecules into separate fatty acids and glycerol again. Fatty acids are divided into two kinds: saturated and unsaturated fatty acids depending on how much hydrogen they contain. The fat found in animals bodies and in dairy products contains mainly saturated fatty acids and tends to be solid at room temperature. Fish and poultry fats and plant oils contain mostly unsaturated fatty acids and are more liquid at room temperature.

Phospholipids are lipids that contain a phosphate group. They are important in the plasma membrane of the cell.

Proteins

Proteins are the third main group of organic compounds in the cell - in fact if you dried out a cell you would find that about 2/3 of the dry dust you were left with would consist of protein. Like carbohydrates and fats, proteins contain C, H and O but they all also contain nitrogen. Many also contain sulphur and phosphorus.

In the cell, proteins are an important part of the plasma membrane of the cell, but their most essential role is as enzymes. These are molecules that act as biological catalysts and are necessary for biochemical reactions to proceed. Protein is also found as keratin in the skin, feathers and hair, in muscles, as well as in antibodies and some hormones.

Proteins are built up of long chains of smaller molecules called amino acids. There are 20 common types of amino acid and different numbers of these arranged in different orders create the multitude of individual proteins that exist in an animal's body.

Long chains of amino acids often link with other amino acid chains and the resulting protein molecule may twist, spiral and fold up to make a complex 3-dimensional shape. As an example, see the diagram of the protein lysozyme below. Believe it or not, this is a small and relatively simple protein.

t is this shape that determines how proteins behave in cells, particularly when they are acting as enzymes. If for any reason this shape is altered, the protein stops working. This is what happens if proteins are heated or put in a solution that is too acidic or alkaline. Think what happens to the "white"" of an egg when it is cooked. The "white" contains the protein albumin, which is changed or "denatured" permanently by cooking. The catastrophic effect that heat has on enzymes is one of the reasons animals die if exposed to high temperatures.

In the animal's diet, proteins are found in meat (muscle), dairy products, seeds, nuts and legumes like soya. When the enzymes in the gut digest proteins they break them down into the separate amino acids, which are small enough to be absorbed into the blood.

Classification

Classification is the process used by scientists to make sense of the 1.5 million or so different kinds of living organisms on the planet. It does this by describing, naming and placing them in different groups. As veterinary nurses you are mainly concerned with the Animal Kingdom but don't forget that animals rely on the Plant Kingdom for food to survive. Also many diseases that animals are affected by are members of the other Kingdoms -- fungi, bacteria and single celled animals.

Naming And Classifying Animals

There are more than 1.5 million different kinds of living organism on Earth ranging from small and simple bacteria to large, complex mammals. From the earliest time that humans have studied the natural world they have named these living organisms and placed them in different groups on the basis of their similarities and differences.

Naming Animals

Of course we know what a cat, a dog and a whale are but, in some situations using the common names for animals can be confusing. Problems arise because people in different countries, and even sometimes in the same country, have different common names for the same animals. For example a cat can be a chat, a Katze, gato, katt, or a moggie, depending on which language you use. To add to the confusion sometimes the same name is used for different animals. For example, the name 'gopher' is used for ground squirrels, rodents (pocket gophers), for moles and in the south-eastern United States for a turtle. This is the reason why all animals have been given an official scientific or binomial name. Unfortunately these names are always in Latin. For example:

- Common rat: Rattus rattus
- Human: Homo sapiens
- Domestic cat: Felis domesticus
- Domestic dog: Canis familiaris

As you can see from the above there are certain rules about writing scientific names:

- They always have 2 parts to them.
- The first part is the genus name and is always written with a capital first letter.
- The second name is the species name and is always written in lower case.
- The name is always underlined or printed in italics.

The first time you refer to an organism you should write the whole name in full. If you need to keep referring to the same organism you can then abbreviate the genus name to just the initial. Thus "Canis familiaris" becomes "C. familiaris" the second and subsequent times you refer to it.

Classification of Living Organisms

To make some sense of the multitude of living organisms they have been placed in different groups. The method that has been agreed by biologists for doing this is called the classification system. The system is based on the assumption that the process of evolution has, over the millennia, brought about slow changes that have converted simple one-celled organisms to complex multi-celled ones and generated the earth's incredible diversity of life forms. The classification system attempts to reflect the evolutionary relationships between organisms.

Initially this classification was based only on the appearance of the organism. However, the development of new techniques has advanced our scientific knowledge. The light microscope and later the electron microscope have enabled us to view the smallest structures, and now techniques for comparing DNA have begun to clarify still further the relationships between organisms. In the light of the advances in knowledge the classification has undergone numerous revisions over time.

At present most biologists divide the living world into 5 kingdoms, namely:

- bacteria
- protists
- fungi
- plants
- animal

We are concerned here almost entirely with the Animal Kingdom. However, we must not forget that bacteria, protists, and fungi cause many of the serious diseases that affect animals, and all animals rely either directly or indirectly on the plant world for their nourishment.

The Animal Kingdom

So what are animals? If we were suddenly confronted with an animal we had never seen in our lives before, how would we know it was not a plant or even a fungus? We all intuitively know part of the answer to this.

Animals

- eat organic material (plants or other animals)
- move to find food
- take the food into their bodies and then digest it
- and most reproduce by fertilizing eggs by sperm

If you were tempted to add that animals are furry, run around on four legs and give birth to young that they feed on milk you were thinking only of mammals and forgetting temporarily that frogs, snakes and crocodiles, birds as well as fish, are also animals.

These are all members of the group called the vertebrates (or animals with a backbone) and mammals make up only about 8% of this group. The diagram on the next page shows the percentage of the different kinds of vertebrates. However, the term animal includes much more than just the Vertebrates. In fact this group makes up only a very small portion of all animals. Take a look at the diagram below, which shows the size of the different groups of animals in the Animal Kingdom as proportions of the total number of different animal species. Notice the small size of the segment representing vertebrates! All the other animals in the Animal Kingdom are animals with no backbone, or invertebrates. This includes the worms, sea anemones, starfish, snails, crabs, spiders and insects. As more than 90% of the invertebrates are insects, no wonder people worry that insects may take over the world one day!

The Classification of Vertebrates

As we have seen above the Vertebrates are divided into 5 groups or classes namely:

- Fish
- Amphibia (frogs and toads)
- Reptiles (snakes and crocodiles)
- Birds
- Mammals

These classes are all based on similarities. For instance all mammals have a similar skeleton, hair on their bodies, are warm bodied and suckle their young.

The class Mammalia (the mammals) contains 3 subclasses:

- Duck billed platypus and the spiny anteater
- Marsupials (animals like the kangaroo with pouches)
- True mammals (with a placenta)

Within the subclass containing the true mammals, there are groupings called orders that contain mammals that are more closely similar or related, than others. Examples of six mammalian orders are given below:

- Rodents (Rodentia) (rats and mice)
- Carnivores (Carnivora) (cats, dogs, bears and seals)
- Even-toed grazers (Artiodactyla) (pigs, sheep, cattle, antelopes)
- Odd-toed grazers (Perissodactyla) (horses, donkeys, zebras)
- Marine mammals (Cetacea) (whales, sea cows)
- Primates (monkeys, apes, humans)

Within each order there are various families. For example within the carnivore mammals are the families:

- Canidae (dog-like carnivores)

- Felidae (cat-like carnivores)

Even at this point it is possible to find groupings that are more closely related than others. These groups are called genera (singular genus). For instance within the cat family Felidae is the genus Felis containing the cats, as well as genera containing panthers, lynxes, and sabre toothed tigers!

The final groups within the system are the species. The definition of a species is a group of animals that can mate successfully and produce fertile offspring. This means that all domestic cats belong to the species Felis domesticus, because all breeds of cat whether Siamese, Manx or ordinary House hold cat can cross breed. However, domestic cats can not mate successfully with lions, tigers or jaguars, so these are placed in separate species, e.g. Felis leo, Felis tigris and Felis onca.

Even within the same species, there can be animals with quite wide variations in appearance that still breed successfully. We call these different breeds, races or varieties. For example there are many different breeds of dogs from Dalmatian to Chihuahua and of cats, from Siamese to Manx and domestic short-hairs, but all can cross breed. Often these breeds have been produced by selective breeding but varieties can arise in the wild when groups of animals are separated by a mountain range or sea and have developed different characteristics over long periods of time.

- To summarise, the classification system consists of:
- The Animal Kingdom which is divided into
- Phyla which are divided into
- Classes which are divided into
- Orders which are divided into
- Families which are divided into
- Genera which are divided into
- Species.

3

THE CELL

The cell is the basic building block of living organisms. Bacteria and the parasite that causes malaria consist of single cells, while plants and animals are made up of trillions of cells. Most cells are spherical or cube shaped but some are a range of different shapes

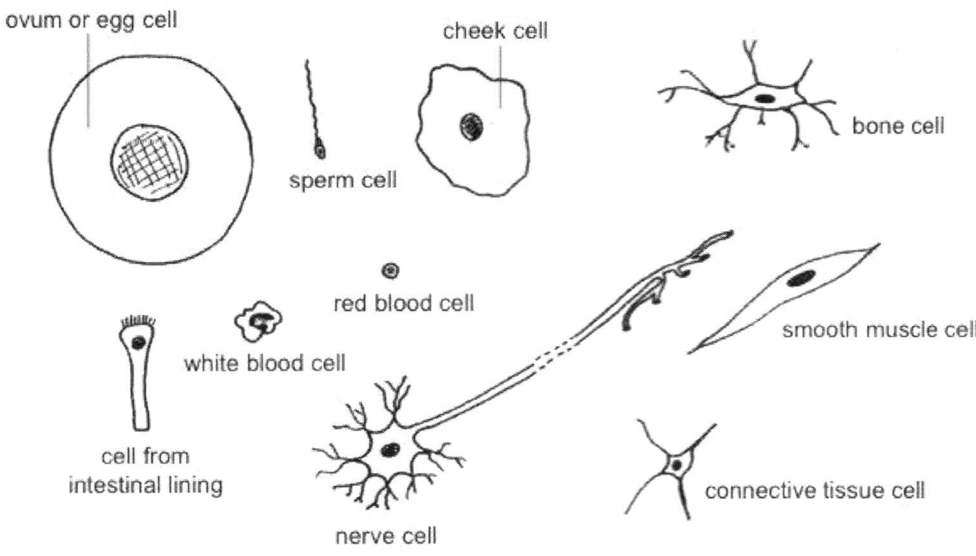

Fig. 3.1 A variety of animal cells

The Cell

Most cells are so small that a microscope is needed to see them, although a few cells, e.g. the ostrich's egg, are so large that they could make a meal for several people.

A normal cell is about 0.02 of a millimetre (0.02mm) in diameter. (Small distances like this are normally expressed in micrometres or microns (μm). Note there are 1000 μms in every mm).

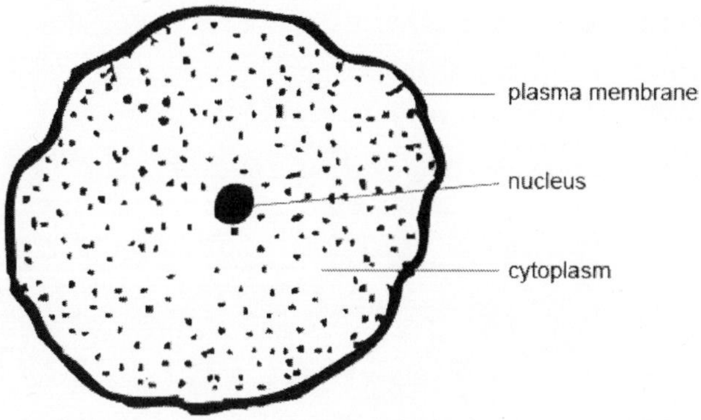

Fig. 3.2 An animal cell

When you look at a typical animal cell with a light microscope it seems quite simple with only a few structures visible.

Three main parts can be seen:

- an outer cell membrane (plasma membrane),
- an inner region called the cytoplasm and
- the nucleus

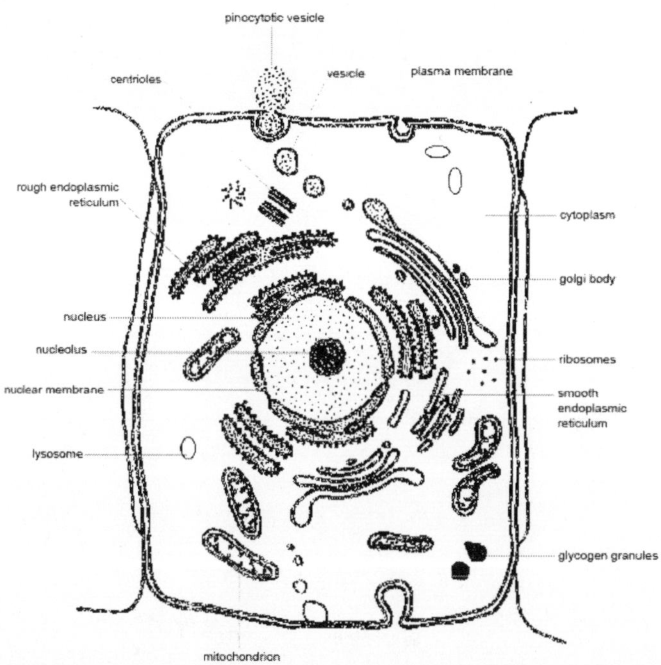

Fig: 3.3 An animal cell as seen with an electron microscope

However, when you use an electron microscope to increase the magnification many thou- sands of times you see that these seemingly simple structures are incredibly complex, each with its own specialized function. For example the plasma membrane is seen to be a dou- ble layer and the cytoplasm contains many special structures called organelles (meaning little organs) which are described below. A drawing of the cell as seen with an electron microscope.

The Plasma Membrane

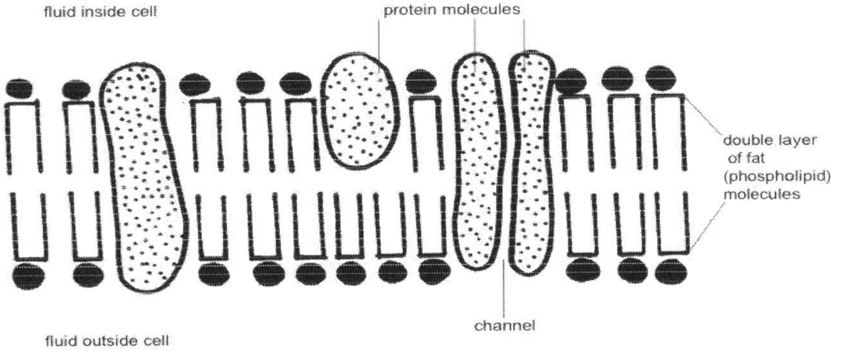

Fig: 3.4 The structure of the plasma membrane

The thin plasma membrane surrounds the cell, separating its contents from the surroundings and controlling what enters and leaves the cell. The plasma membrane is composed of two main molecules,phospholipids(fats) and proteins. The phospholipids are arranged in a double layer with the large protein molecules dotted about in the membrane. Some of the protein molecules form tiny channels in the membrane while others help transport substances from one side of the membrane to the other.

How substances move across the Plasma Membrane

Substances need to pass through the membrane to enter or leave the cell and they do so in a number of ways. Some of these processes require no energy i.e. they are passive, while others require energy i.e. they are active .

Passive processes include: a) diffusion and b) osmosis, while active processes include: c) active transport, d) phagocytosis, e) pinocytosis and f) exocytosis. These will be described below.

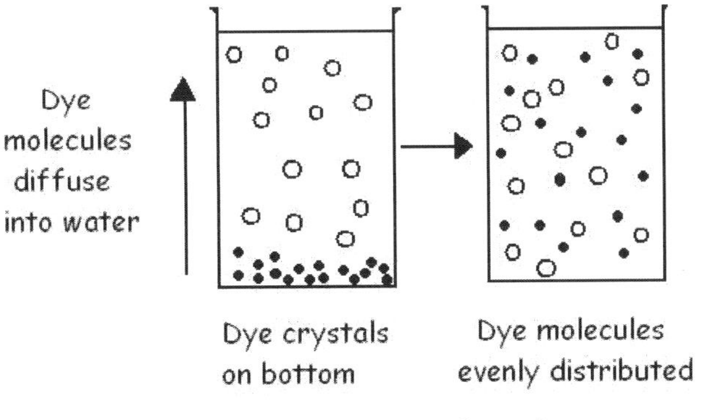

Fig. 3.5 Diffusion in a liquid

(a) Diffusion

Although you may not know it, you are already familiar with the process of diffusion. It is diffusion that causes a smell (expensive perfume or smelly socks) in one part of the room to gradually move through the room so it can be smelt on the other side. Diffusion occurs in the air and in liquids.

Diagram 3.5 shows what happens when a few crystals of a dark purple dye called potassium permanganate are dropped into a beaker of water. The dye molecules diffuse into the water moving from high to low concentrations so they become evenly distributed throughout the beaker.

In the body, diffusion causes molecules that are in a high concentration on one side of the cell membrane to move across the membrane until they are present in equal concentrations on both sides. It takes place because all molecules have an in-built vibration that causes them to move and collide until they are evenly distributed. It is an absolutely natural process that requires no added energy.

Small molecules like oxygen, carbon dioxide, water and ammonia as well as fats, diffuse directly through the double fat layer of the membrane. The small molecules named above as well as a variety of charged particles (ions) also diffuse through the protein-lined channels. Larger molecules like glucose attach to a carrier molecule that aids their diffusion through the membrane. This is called facilitated diffusion .

In the animal's body diffusion is important for moving oxygen and carbon dioxide between the lungs and the blood, for moving digested food molecules from the gut into the blood and for the removal of waste products from the cell.

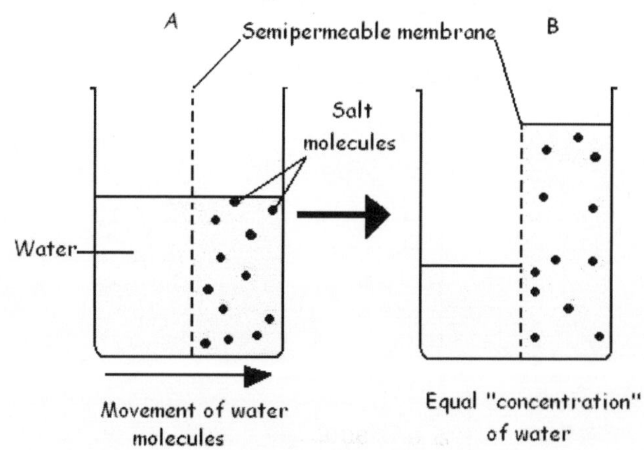

Fig: 3.6 Osmosis

(b) Osmosis

Although the word may be unfamiliar, you are almost certainly acquainted with the effects of osmosis. It is osmosis that plumps out dried fruit when you soak it before making a fruit cake or makes that wizened old carrot look almost like new when you soak it in water. Osmosis is in fact the diffusion of water across a membrane that allows water across but not larger molecules. This kind of membrane is called a semi-permeable membrane .

Take a look at side A of diagram 3.6. It shows a container divided into two parts by an artificial semi-permeable membrane. Water is poured into one part while a solution containing salt is poured into the other part. Water can cross the membrane but the salt cannot. The water crosses the semi-permeable membrane by diffusion until there is an equal amount of water on both sides of the membrane. The effect of this would be to make the salt solution more diluted and cause the level of the liquid in the right-hand side of the container to rise so it looked like side B of diagram 3.6. This movement of water across the semi-permeable membrane is called osmosis. It is a completely natural process that requires no outside energy.

Although it would be difficult to do in practice, imagine that you could now take a plunger and push down on the fluid in the right-hand side of container B so that it flowed back across the semi-permeable membrane until the level of fluid on both sides was equal again. If you could measure the pressure required to do this, this would be equal to the osmotic

pressure of the salt solution. (This is a rather advanced concept at this stage but you will meet this term again when you study fluid balance later in the course).

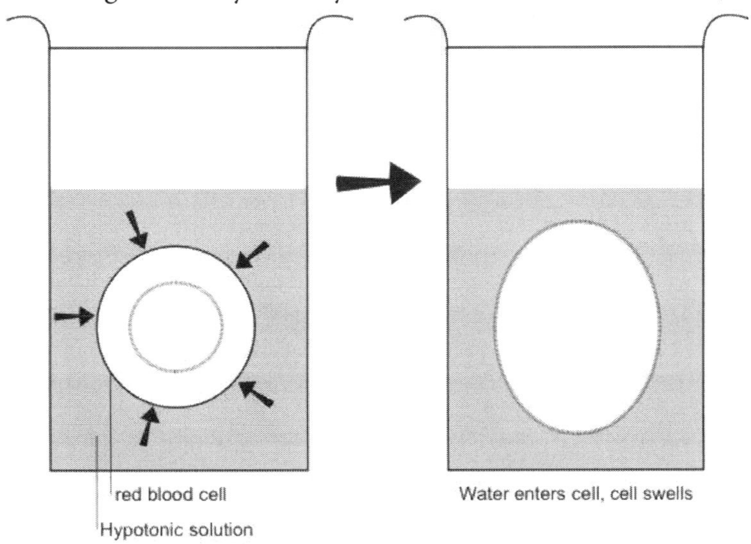

Fig. 3.7 Osmosis in red cells placed in a hypotonic solution

The plasma membrane of cells acts as a semi-permeable membrane. If red blood cells, for example, are placed in water, the water crosses the membrane to make the amount of water on both sides of it equal (see diagram 3.7). This means that the water moves into the cell causing it to swell. This can occur to such an extent that the cell actually bursts to release its contents. This bursting of red blood cells is called haemolysis . In a situation such as this when the solution on one side of a semi-permeable membrane has a lower concentration than that on the other side, the first solution is said to be hypotonic to the second.

Now think what would happen if red blood cells were placed in a salt solution that has a higher salt concentration than the solution within the cells (see diagram 3.8). Such a bathing solution is called a hypertonic solution. In this situation the "concentration" of water within the cells would be higher than that outside the cells. Osmosis (diffusion of water) would then occur from the inside of the cells to the outside solution, causing the cells to shrink.

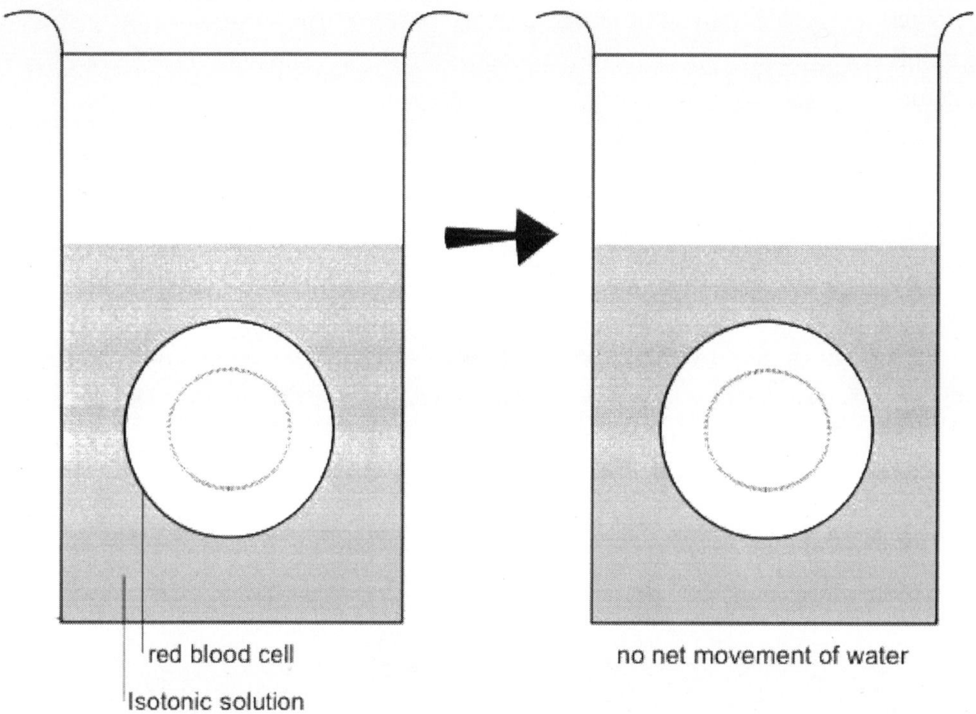

Fig. 3.8 Red cells placed in an isotonic solution

A solution that contains 0.9% salt has the same concentration as body fluids and the solution within red cells. Cells placed in such a solution would neither swell nor shrink (see diagram 3.9). This solution is called an isotonic solution. This strength of salt solution is often called normal saline and is used when replacing an animal's body fluids or when cells like red blood cells have to be suspended in fluid.

Remember - osmosis is a special kind of diffusion. It is the diffusion of water molecules across a semi-permeable membrane. It is a completely passive process and requires no energy.

Sometimes it is difficult to remember which way the water molecules move. Although it is not strictly true in a biological sense, many students use the phrase "SALT SUCKS" to help them remember which way water moves across the membrane when there are two solutions of different salt concentrations on either side.

As we have seen water moves in and out of the cell by osmosis. All water movement from the intestine into the blood system and between the blood capillaries and the fluid around the cells (tissue or extra cellular fluid) takes place by osmosis. Osmosis is also important in the production of concentrated urine by the kidney.

(c) Active transport

When a substance is transported from a low concentration to a high concentration i.e. uphill against the concentration gradient, energy has to be used. This is called active transport

Active transport is important in maintaining different concentrations of the ions sodium and potassium on either side of the nerve cell membrane. It is also important for removing valuable molecules such as glucose, amino acids and sodium ions from the urine.

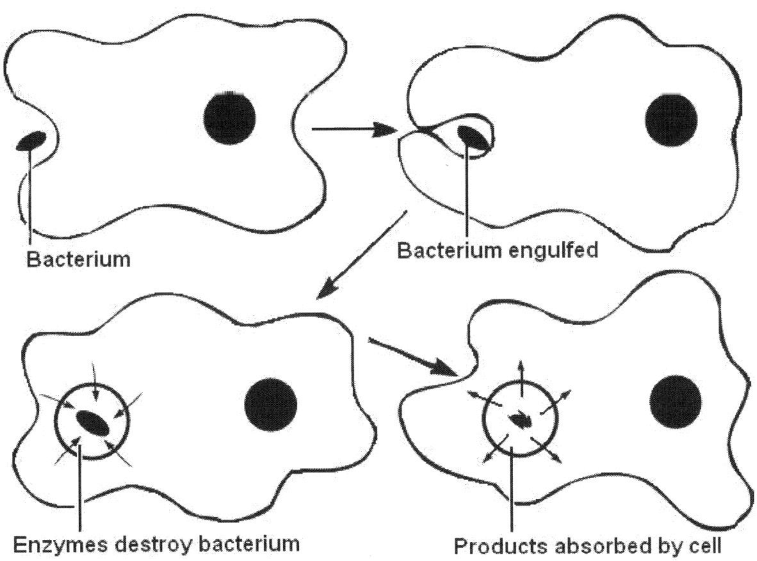

Fig. 3.9 Phagocytosis

(d) Phagocytosis

Phagocytosis is sometimes called "cell eating". It is a process that requires energy and is used by cells to move solid particles like bacteria across the plasma membrane. Finger-like projections from the plasma membrane surround the bacteria and engulf them as shown in diagram 3.10. Once within the cell, enzymes produced by the lysosomes of the cell (described later) destroy the bacteria.

The destruction of bacteria and other foreign substance by white blood cells by the process of phagocytosis is a vital part of the defense mechanisms of the body.

(e) Pinocytosis

Pinocytosis or "cell drinking" is a very similar process to phagocytosis but is used by cells to move fluids across the plasma membrane. Most cells carry out pinocytosis (note the pinocytotic vesicle in diagram 3.3).

(f) Exocytosis

The Cytoplasm

Exocytosis is the process by means of which substances formed in the cell are moved through the plasma membrane into the fluid outside the cell (or extra-cellular fluid). It occurs in all cells but is most important in secretory cells (e.g. cells that produce digestive enzymes) and nerve cells.

The Cytoplasm

Within the plasma membrane is the cytoplasm . It consists of a clear jelly-like fluid called the a) cytosol or intracellular fluid in which b) cell inclusions , c) organelles and d) microfilaments and microtubules are found.

(a) Cytosol

The cytosol consists mainly of water in which various molecules are dissolved or suspended. These molecules include proteins, fats and carbohydrates as well as sodium, potassium, calcium and chloride ions. Many of the reactions that take place in the cell occur in the cytosol.

(b) Cell inclusions

These are large particles of fat, glycogen and melanin that have been produced by the cell. They are often large enough to be seen with the light microscope. For example the cells of adipose tissue (as in the insulating fat layer under the skin) contain fat that takes up most of the cell.

(c) Organelles

Organelles are the "little organs" of the cell - like the heart, kidney and liver are the organs of the body. They are structures with characteristic appearances and specific "jobs" in the cell. Most can not be seen with the light microscope and so it was only when the electron microscope was developed that they were discovered. The main organelles in the cell are the ribosomes, endoplasmic reticulum, mitochondrion, Golgi complex and lysosomes

A cell containing these organelles as seen with the electron microscope is shown in diagram 3.3.

Ribosomes

Ribosomes are tiny spherical organelles that make proteins by joining amino acids to- gether. Many ribosomes are found free in the cytosol, while others are attached to the rough endoplasmic reticulum.

Endoplasmic reticulum

The endoplasmic reticulum (ER) is a network of membranes that form channels throughout the cytoplasm from the nucleus to the plasma membrane. Various molecules are made in the ER and transported around the cell in its channels. There are two types of ER: smooth ER and rough ER.

Smooth ER is where the fats in the cell are made and in some cells, where chemicals like alcohol, pesticides and carcinogenic molecules are inactivated.

The Rough ER has ribosomes attached to its surface. The function of the Rough ER is therefore to make proteins that are modified stored and transported by the ER

Mitochondria

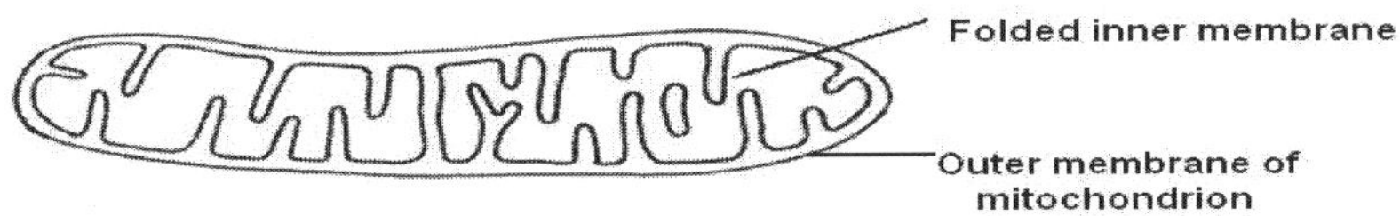

Fig. 3.10 A mitochondrion

Mitochondria (singular mitochondrion) are oval or rod shaped organelles scattered throughout the cytoplasm. They consist of two membranes, the inner one of which is folded to increase its surface area. (Diagram 3.10)

Mitochondria are the "power stations" of the cell. They make energy by "burning" food molecules like glucose. This process is called cellular respiration . The reaction requires oxygen and produces carbon dioxide which is a waste product. The process is very com- plex and takes place in a large number of steps but the overall word equation for cellular respiration is-

Glucose + oxygen = carbon dioxide + water + energy

Note that cellular respiration is different from respiration or breathing. Breathing is the means by which air is drawn into and expelled from the lungs. Breathing is necessary to supply the cells with the oxygen required by the mitochondria and to remove the carbon dioxide produced as a waste product of cellular respiration.

Active cells like muscle, liver, kidney and sperm cells have large numbers of mitochondria.

Golgi Apparatus

The Nucleus

The Golgi bodies in a cell together make up the Golgi apparatus . Golgi bodies are found near the nucleus and consist of flattened membranes stacked on top of each other rather like a pile of plates. The Golgi apparatus modifies and sorts the proteins and fats made by the ER, then surrounds them in a membrane as vesicles so they can be moved to other parts of the cell.

Lysosomes

Lysosomes are large vesicles that contain digestive enzymes. These break down bacteria and other substances that are brought into the cell by phagocytosis or pinocytosis. They also digest worn-out or damaged organelles, the components of which can then be recycled by the cell to make new structures.

(d) Microfilaments And Microtubules

Some cells can move and change shape and organelles and chemicals are moved around the cell. Threadlike structures called microfilaments and microtubules that can contract are responsible for this movement.

These structures also form the projections from the plasma membrane known as flagella (singular flagellum) as in the sperm tail, and cilia found lining the respiratory tract and used to remove mucus that has trapped dust particles.

Microtubules also form the pair of cylindrical structures called centrioles found near the nucleus. These help organise the spindle used in cell division.

The Nucleus

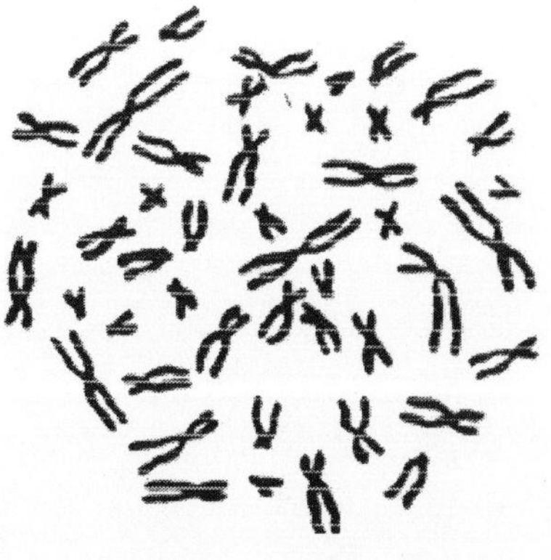

Fig. 3.11 A full set of human chromosomes

The nucleus is the largest structure in a cell and can be seen with the light microscope. It is a spherical or oval body that contains the chromosomes . The nucleus controls the development and activity of the cell. Most cells contain a nucleus although mature red blood cells have lost theirs during development and some muscle cells have several nuclei.

A double membrane similar in structure to the plasma membrane surrounds the nucleus (now called the nuclear envelope). Pores in this nuclear membrane allow communication between the nucleus and the cytoplasm.

Within the nucleus one or more spherical bodies of darker material can be seen, even with the light microscope. These are called nucleoli and are made of RNA. Their role is to make new ribosomes.

Chromosomes

Inside the nucleus are the chromosomes which:

- contain DNA;
- control the activity of the cell;
- are transmitted from cell to cell when cells divide;
- are passed to a new individual when sex cells fuse together in sexual reproduction.

In cells that are not dividing the chromosomes are very long and thin and appear as dark grainy material. They become visible just before a cell divides when they shorten and thicken and can then be counted.

The number of chromosomes in the cells of different species varies but is constant in the cells of any one species (e.g. horses have 64 chromosomes, cats have 38 and humans 46). Chromosomes occur in pairs (i.e. 32 pairs in the horse nucleus and 19 in that of the cat). Members of each pair are identical in length and shape and if you look carefully, you may be able to see some of the pairs in the human set of chromosomes.

Cell Division

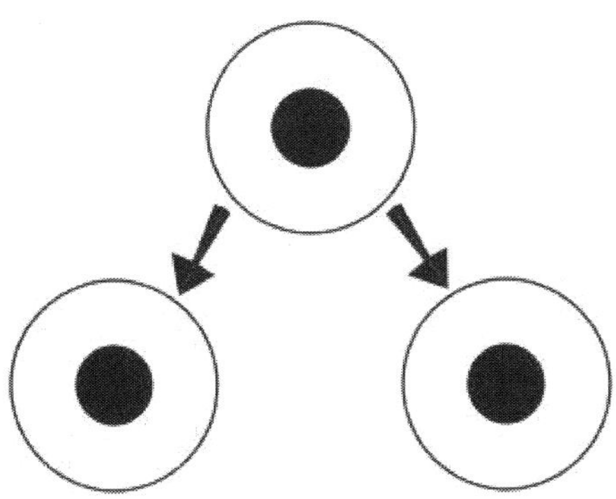

Fig. 3.12 Division by mitosis results in 2 new cells identical to each other and to parent cell

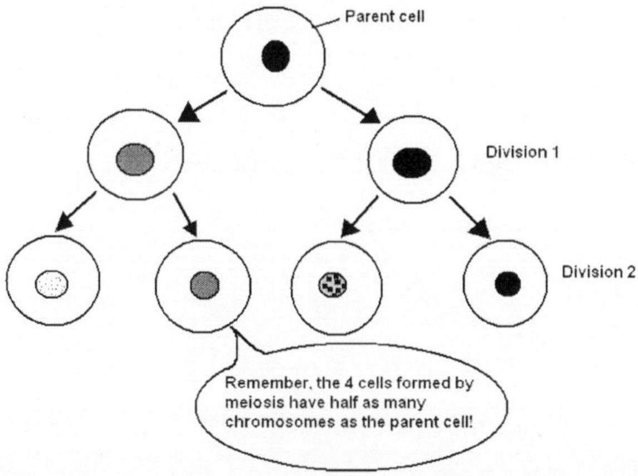

Fig. 3.13 Division by meiosis results in 4 new cells that are genetically different to each other

Cells divide when an animal grows, when its body repairs an injury and when it produces sperm and eggs (or ova). There are two types of cell division: Mitosis and meiosis .

Mitosis . This is the cell division that occurs when an animal grows and when tissues are repaired or replaced. It produces two new cells (daughter cells) each with a full set of chromosomes that are identical to each other and to the parent cell. All the cells of an animal's body therefore contain identical DNA.

Meiosis. This is the cell division that produces the ova and sperm necessary for sexual reproduction. It only occurs in the ovary and testis.

The most important function of meiosis it to halve the number of chromosomes so that when the sperm fertilises the ovum the normal number is regained. Body cells with the full set of chromosomes are called diploid cells, while gametes (sperm and ova) with half the chromosomes are called haploid cells.

Meiosis is a more complex process than mitosis as it involves two divisions one after the other and the four cells produced are all genetically different from each other and from the parent cell.

This fact that the cells formed by meiosis are all genetically different from each other and from the parent cell can be seen in litters of kittens where all the members of the litter are different from each other as well as being different from the parents although they display characteristics of both.

4

BODY ORGANISATION

In this chapter, the way the cells of the body are organised into different tissues is described. You will find out how these tissues are arranged into organs, and how the organs form systems such as the digestive system and the reproductive system. Also in this chapter, the important concept of homeostasis is defined. You are also introduced to those pesky things directional terms.

4.1 OBJECTIVES

After completing this section, you should know:

- the "Mrs Gren" characteristics of living organisms
- what a tissue is
- four basic types of tissues, their general function and where they are found in the body
- the basic organisation of the body of vertebrates including the main body cavities and the location of the following major organs: thorax, heart, lungs, thymus, abdomen, liver, stomach, spleen, intestines, kidneys, sperm ducts, ovaries, uterus, cervix, vagina, urinary bladder
- the 11 body systems
- what homeostasis is
- directional terms including dorsal, ventral, caudal, cranial, medial, lateral, proximal, distal, rostral, palmar and plantar. Plus transverse and longitudinal sections

4.2 The Organisation of Animal Bodies

Living organisms move, feed, respire (burn food to make energy), grow, sense their envi- ronment, excrete and reproduce. These seven characteristics are sometimes summarized by the words "MRS GREN". functions of:

- Movement R espiration S ensitivity G rowth
- Reproduction
- Excretion
- Nutrition

Living organisms are made from cells which are organised into tissues and these are them- selves combined to form organs and systems.

Skin cells, muscle cells, skeleton cells and nerve cells, for example. These different types of cells are not just scattered around randomly but similar cells that perform the same function are arranged in groups. These collections of similar cells are known as tissues .

There are four main types of tissues in animals. These are:

- Epithelial tissues that form linings, coverings and glands,
- Connective tissues for transport and support
- Muscle tissues for movement and
- Nervous tissues for carrying messages.

Epithelial Tissues

Epithelium (plural epithelia) is tissue that covers and lines. It covers an organ or lines a tube or space in the body. There are several different types of epithelium, distinguished by the different shapes of the cells and whether they consist of only a single layer of cells or several layers of cells.

Simple Epithelia - with a single layer of cells

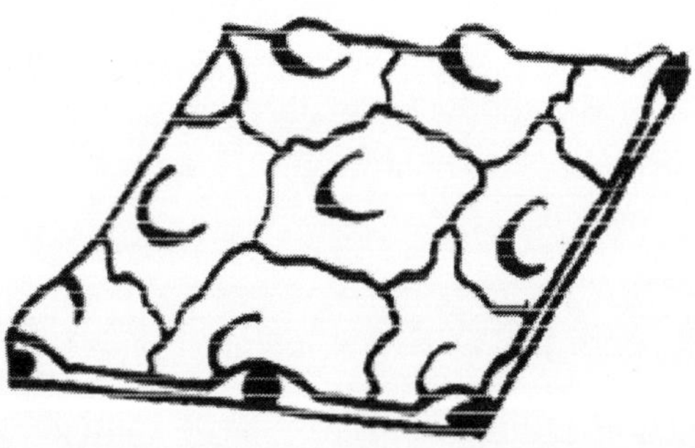

FIG. 4.1 SQUAMOUS EPITHELIUM

Squamous epithelium

Squamous epithelium consists of a single layer of flattened cells that are shaped rather like 'crazy paving'. It is found lining the heart, blood vessels, lung alveoli and body cavities. Its thinness allows molecules to diffuse across readily.

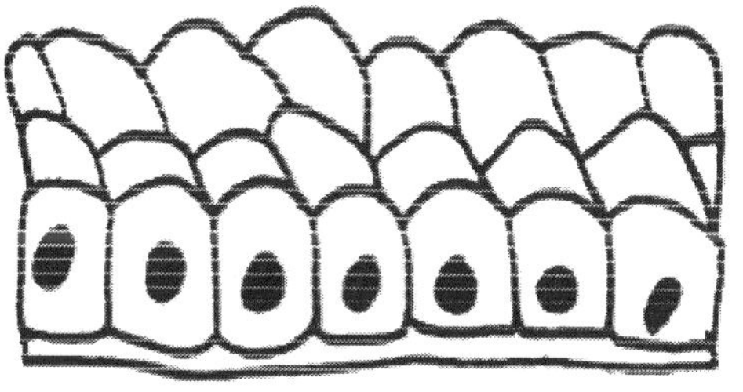

Fig. 4.2 Cuboidal epithelium

Cuboidal epithelium

Cuboidal epithelium consists of a single layer of cube shaped cells. It is rare in the body but is found lining kidney tubules. Molecules pass across it by diffusion, osmosis and active transport.

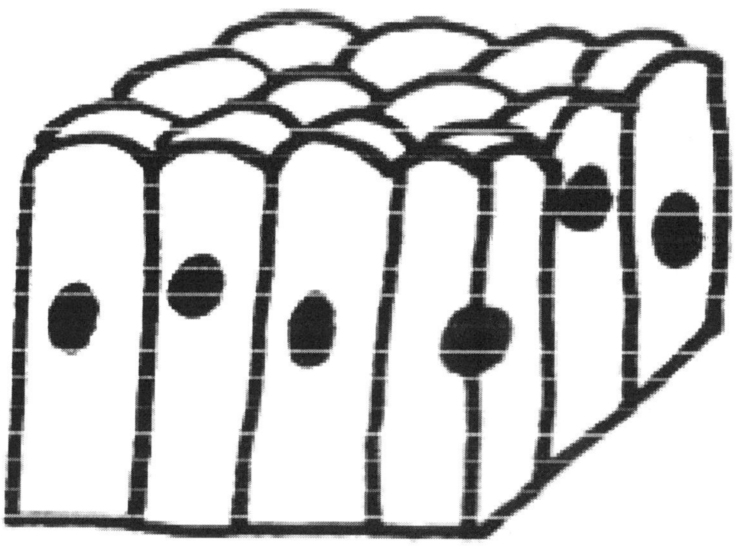

Fig. 4.3 Columnar epithelium

Columnar epithelium

Columnar epithelium consists of column shaped cells. It is found lining the gut from the stomach to the anus. Digested food products move across it into the blood stream.

Columnar epithelium with cilia

Columnar epithelium with cilia on the free surface (also known as the apical side of the cell) lines the respiratory tract, fallopian tubes and uterus (see diagram 4.4). The cilia beat rhythmically to transport particles.

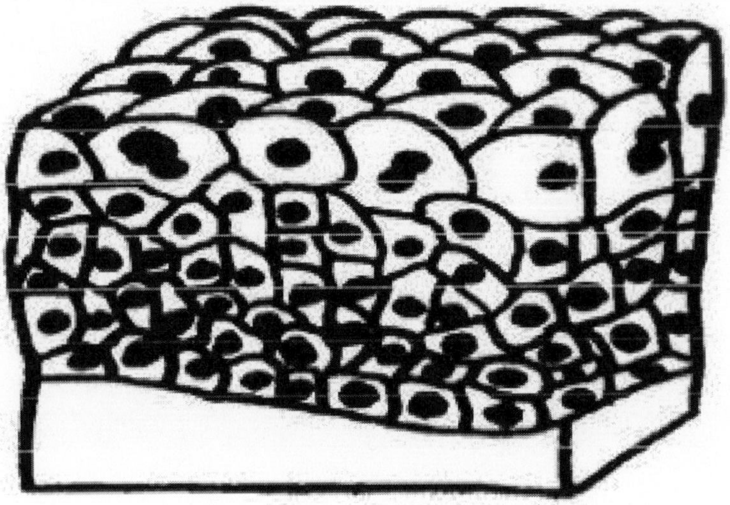

Fig. 4.4 Transitional epithelium

Transitional epithelium - with a variable number of layers

The cells in transitional epithelium can move over one another allowing it to stretch. It is found in the wall of the bladder.

Stratified epithelia - with several layers of cells.

Epithelia with several layers of cells are found where toughness and resistance to abrasion are needed.

Stratified squamous epithelium

Stratified squamous epithelium has many layers of flattened cells. It is found lining the mouth, cervix and vagina. Cells at the base divide and push up the cells above them and cells at the top are worn or pushed off the surface. This type of epithelium protects underlying layers and repairs itself rapidly if damaged.

Keratinised stratified squamous epithelium

Keratinised stratified squamous epithelium has a tough waterproof protein called keratin deposited in the cells. It forms the skin found covering the outer surface of mammals.

Connective Tissues

Blood, bone, tendons, cartilage, fibrous connective tissue and fat (adipose) tissue are all classed as connective tissues. They are tissues that are used for supporting the body or transporting substances around the body. They also consist of three parts: they all have cells suspended in a ground substance or matrix and most have fibres running through it.

Blood

Blood consists of a matrix - plasma, with several types of cells and cell fragments suspended in it. The fibres are only evident in blood that has clotted. Blood will be described in detail in chapter 8.

Lymph

Lymph is similar in composition to blood plasma with various types of white blood cell floating in it. It flows in lymphatic vessels.

Connective tissue 'proper'

Connective tissue 'proper' consists of a jelly-like matrix with a dense network of collagen and elastic fibres and various cells embedded in it. There are various different forms of 'proper' connective tissue.

Loose connective tissue

Loose connective tissue is a sticky whitish substance that fills the spaces between organs. It is found in the dermis of the skin.

Dense connective tissue

Dense connective tissue contains lots of thick fibres and is very strong. It forms tendons, ligaments and heart valves and covers bones and organs like the kidney and liver.

Adipose tissue

Adipose tissue consists of cells filled with fat. It forms the fatty layer under the dermis of the skin, around the kidneys and heart and the yellow marrow of the bones.

Cartilage

Cartilage is the 'gristle' of the meat. It consists of a tough jelly-like matrix with cells suspended in it. It may contain collagen and elastic fibres. It is a flexible but tough tissue and is found at the ends of bones, in the nose, ear and trachea and between the vertebrae.

Bone

Bone consists of a solid matrix made of calcium salts that give it its hardness. Collagen fibres running through it give it its strength. Bone cells are found in spaces in the matrix. Two types of bone are found in the skeleton namely spongy and compact bone . They differ in the way the cells and matrix are arranged.

MUSCLE TISSUES

Muscle tissue is composed of cells that contract and move the body. There are three types of muscle tissue:

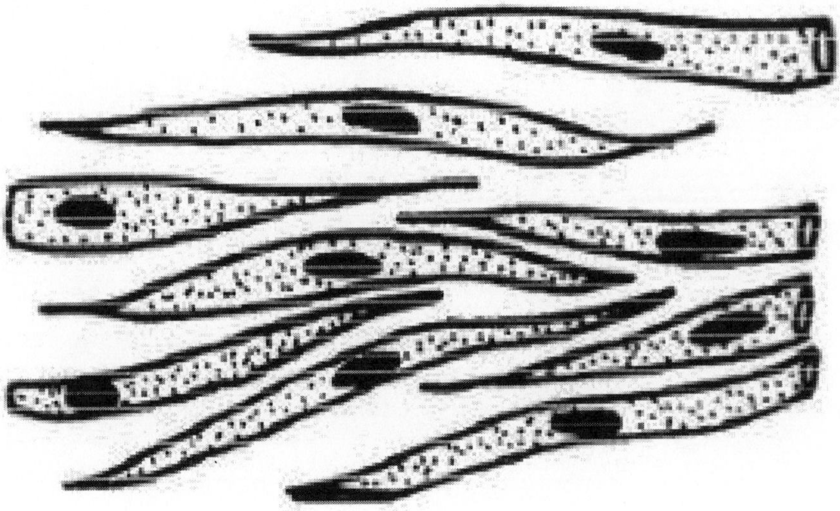

Fig. 4.5 Smooth muscle fibres

SMOOTH MUSCLE

Smooth muscle consists of long and slender cells with a central nucleus (see diagram 4.9). It is found in the walls of blood vessels, airways to the lungs and the gut. It changes the size of the blood vessels and helps move food and fluid along. Contraction of smooth muscle fibres occurs without the conscious control of the animal.

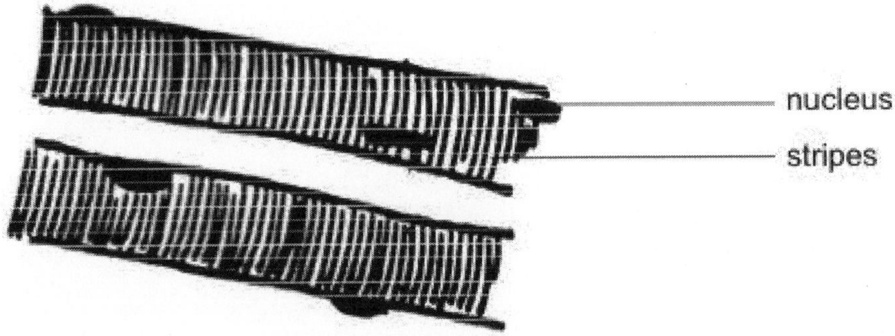

Fig. 4.7 Skeletal muscle fibres

Skeletal muscle

Skeletal muscle (sometimes called striated , striped or voluntary muscle) has striped fibres with alternating light and dark bands. It is attached to bones and is under the voluntary control of the animal (see diagram 4.7).

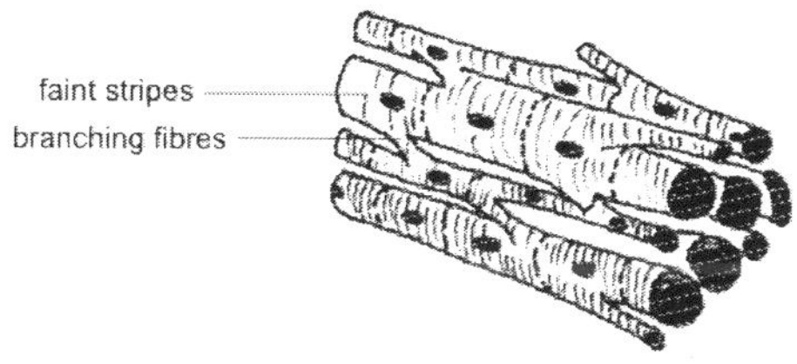

Fig. 4.8 Cardiac muscle fibres

Cardiac muscle

Cardiac muscle is found only in the walls of the heart where it produces the 'heart beat'. Cardiac muscle cells are branched cylinders with central nuclei and faint stripes (see diagram 4.8). Each fibre contracts automatically but the heart beat as a whole is controlled by the pacemaker and the involuntary autonomic nervous system .

NERVOUS TISSUES

Nervous tissue forms the nerves, spinal cord and brain. Nerve cells or neurons consist of a cell body and a long thread or axon that carries the nerve impulse. An insulating sheath of fatty material (myelin) usually surrounds the axon.

Vertebrate Bodies

We are so familiar with animals with backbones (i.e. vertebrates) that it seems rather unnecessary to point out that the body is divided into three sections. There is a well-defined head that contains the brain, the major sense organs and the mouth, a trunk that contains the other organs and a well-developed tail . Other features of vertebrates may be less apparent. For instance, vertebrates that live on the land have developed a flexible neck that is absent in fish where it would be in the way of the gills and interfere with streamlining. Mammals but not other vertebrates have a sheet of muscle called the diaphragm that divides the trunk into the chest region or thorax and the abdomen .

Body Cavities

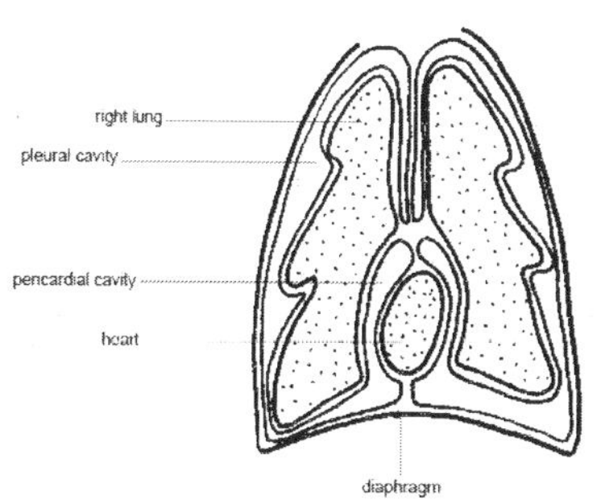

Fig. 4.7 The body cavities

In contrast to many primitive animals, vertebrates have spaces or body cavities that contain the body organs. Most vertebrates have a single body cavity but in mammals the diaphragm divides the main cavity into a thoracic and an abdominal cavity . In the thoracic cavity the heart and lungs are surrounded by their own membranes so that cavities are created around the heart - the pericardial cavity , and around the lungs – the pleural cavity (see diagram 4.9).

Organs

Just as the various parts of the cell work together to perform the cell's functions and a large number of similar cells make up a tissue, so many different tissues can "cooperate" to form an organ that performs a particular function. For example, connective tissues, epithelial tissues, muscle tissue and nervous tissue combine to make the organ that we call the stomach. In turn the stomach combines with other organs like the intestines, liver and pancreas to form the digestive system (see diagram 4.14).

Generalised Plan of the Mammalian Body

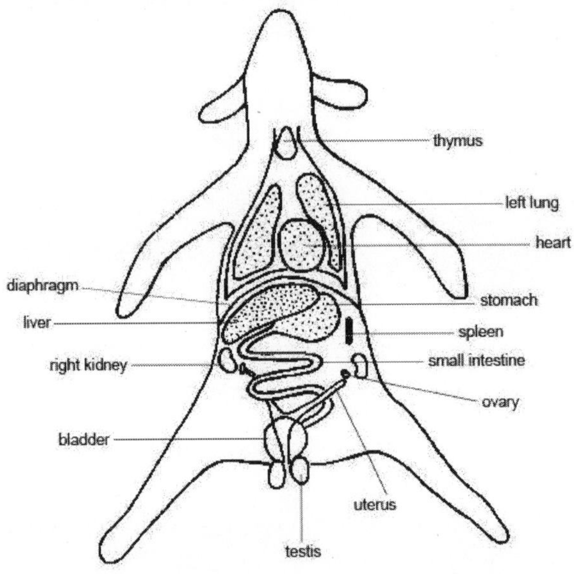

Fig. 4.10 The main organs of the vertebrate body

At this point it would be a good idea to make yourself familiar with the major organs and their positions in the body of a mammal like the rabbit. Diagram 4.10 shows the main body organs.

Body Systems

Organs do not work in isolation but function in cooperation with other organs and body structures to bring about the MRS GREN functions necessary to keep an animal alive. For example the stomach can only work in conjunction with the mouth and oesophagus (gullet). These provide it with the food it breaks down and digests. It then needs to pass the food on to the intestines etc. for further digestion and absorption. The organs involved with the taking of food into the body, the digestion and absorption of the food and elimination of waste products are collectively known as the digestive system.

THE 11 BODY SYSTEMS

1. Skin

The skin covering the body consists of two layers, the epidermis and dermis . Associated with these layers are hairs, feathers, claws, hoofs, glands and sense organs of the skin.

2. Skeletal System

This can be divided into the bones of the skeleton and the joints where the bones move over each other.

3. Muscular System

The muscles, in conjunction with the skeleton and joints, give the body the ability to move.

4. Cardiovascular System

This is also known as the circulatory system. It consists of the heart, the blood vessels and the blood. It transports substances around the body.

5. Lymphatic System

This system is responsible for collecting and "cleaning" the fluid that leaks out of the blood vessels. This fluid is then returned to the blood system. The lymphatic system also makes antibodies that protect the body from invasion by bacteria etc. It consists of lymphatic vessels, lymph nodes, the spleen and thymus glands.

6. Respiratory System

This is the system involved with bringing oxygen in the air into the body and getting rid of carbon dioxide, which is a waste product of processes that occur in the cell. It is made up of the trachea, bronchi, bronchioles, lungs, diaphragm, ribs and muscles that move the ribs in breathing.

7. Digestive System

This is also known as the gastrointestinal system , alimentary system or gut . It consists of the digestive tube and glands like the liver and pancreas that produce digestive secretions. It is concerned with breaking down the large molecules in foods into smaller ones that can be absorbed into the blood and lymph. Waste material is also eliminated by the digestive system.

8. Urinary System

This is also known as the renal system . It removes waste products from the blood and is made up of the kidneys, ureters and bladder.

9. Reproductive System

This is the system that keeps the species going by making new individuals. It is made up of the ovaries, uterus, vagina and fallopian tubes in the female and the testes with associated glands and ducts in the male.

10. Nervous System

This system coordinates the activities of the body and responses to the environment. It consists of the sense organs (eye, ear, semicircular canals, and organs of taste and smell), the nerves, brain and spinal cord.

11. Endocrine System

This is the system that produces chemical messengers or hormones. It consists of various endocrine glands (ductless glands) that include the pituitary, adrenal, thyroid and pineal glands as well as the testes and ovary.

Homeostasis

All the body systems, except the reproductive system, are involved with keeping the con- ditions inside the animal more or less stable. This is called homeostasis . These constant conditions are essential for the survival and proper functioning of the cells, tissues and or- gans of the body. The skin, for example, has an important role in keeping the temperature of the body constant. The kidneys keep the concentration of salts in the blood within limits and the islets of Langerhans in the pancreas maintain the correct level of glucose in the blood through the hormone insulin. As long as the various body processes remain within normal limits, the body functions properly and is healthy. Once homeostasis is disturbed disease or death may result.

Directional Terms

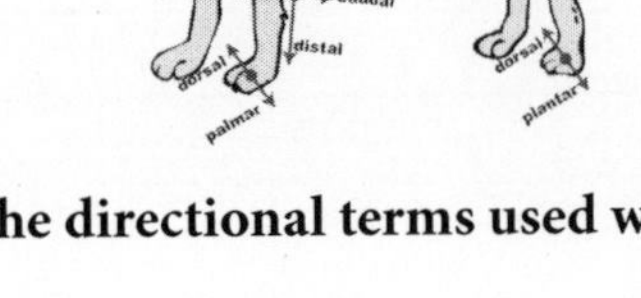

Fig. 4.11 The directional terms used with animals

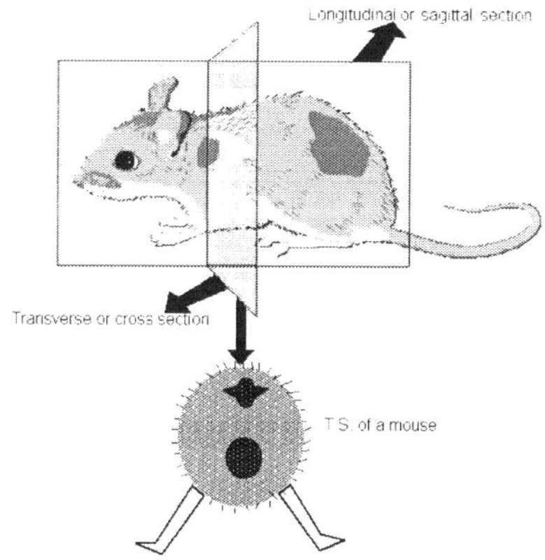

Fig. 4.12 Transverse and longitudinal sections of a mouse

In the following chapters the systems of the body in the list above will be covered one by one. For each one the structure of the organs involved will be described and the way they function will be explained.

In order to describe structures in the body of an animal it is necessary to have a system for describing the position of parts of the body in relation to other parts. For example it may be necessary to describe the position of the liver in relation to the diaphragm, or the heart in relation to the lungs. Certainly if you work further with animals, in a veterinary clinic for example, it will be necessary to be able to accurately describe the position of an injury. The terms used for this are called directional terms .

The most common directional terms are right and left . However, even these are not completely straightforward especially when looking at diagrams of animals. The convention is to show the left side of the animal or organ on the right side of the page. This is the view you would get looking down on an animal lying on its back during surgery or in a post-mortem. Sometimes it is useful to imagine 'getting inside' the animal (so to speak) to check which side is which. The other common and useful directional terms are listed below.

Term	Definition	Example
Dorsal	Nearer the back of the animal	
than	The backbone is dorsal to the	
belly		
Ventral	Nearer the belly of the animal	
than	The breastbone is ventral to	
the heart		
Cranial (or ante-		

rior)	Nearer to the skull than	The diaphragm is cranial to
the stomach		
Caudal (or poste-		
rior)	Nearer to the tail than	The ribs are caudal to the
neck		
Proximal	Closer to the body than (only	
used for structures on limbs)	The shoulder is proximal to	
the elbow		
Distal	Further from the body than (only used for structures on	
limbs)	The ankle is distal to the knee	
Medial	Nearer to the midline than	The bladder is medial to the
hips		
Lateral	Further from the midline than	The ribs are lateral to the
lungs		
Rostral	Towards the muzzle	There are more grey hairs in
the rostral part of the head		
Palmar	The "walking" surface of the	
front paw	There is a small cut on the	
left palmar surface		
Plantar	The "walking" surface of the	
hind paw	The pads are on the plantar	
side of the foot		

Note that we don't use the terms superior and inferior for animals. They are only used to describe the position of structures in the human body (and possibly apes) where the upright posture means some structures are above or superior to others.

In order to look at the structure of some of the parts or organs of the body it may be necessary to cut them open or even make thin slices of them that they can be examined under the microscope. The direction and position of slices or sections through an animal's body have their own terminology.

If an animal or organ is sliced lengthwise this section is called a longitudinal or sagittal section . This is sometimes abbreviated to LS.

If the section is sliced crosswise it is called a transverse or cross section . This is sometimes abbreviated to TS or XS.

5

THE SKIN

The skin is the first of the eleven body systems to be described. Each chapter from now on will cover one body system.

The skin, sometimes known as the Integumentary System is, in fact, the largest organ of the body. It has a complex structure, being composed of many different tissues. It performs many functions that are important in maintaining homeostasis in the body. Probably the most important of these functions is the control of body temperature. The skin also protects the body from physical damage and bacterial invasion. The skin has an array of sense organs which sense the external environment, and also cells which can make vitamin D in sunlight.

The skin is one of the first systems affected when an animal becomes sick so it is important for anyone working with animals to have a sound knowledge of the structure and functioning of the skin so they can quickly recognise signs of disease.

Objectives

After completing this section, you should know:

- the general structure of the skin
- the function of the keratin deposited in the epidermis
- the structure and function of keratin skin structures including calluses, scales, nails, claws, hoofs and horns
- that antlers are not made either of keratin or in the epidermis
- the structure of hairs
- the structure of the different types of feathers and the function of preening
- the general structure and function of sweat, scent, preen and mammary glands

- the basic functions of the skin in sensing stimuli, temperature control and production of vitamin D
- the mechanisms by which the skin regulates body temperature

The Skin

Skin comes in all kinds of textures and forms. There is the dry warty skin of toads and crocodiles, the wet slimy skin of fish and frogs, the hard shell of tortoises and the soft supple skin of snakes and humans. Mammalian skin is covered with hair, that of birds with feathers, and fish and reptiles have scales. Pigment in the skin, hairs or feathers can make the outer surface almost any colour of the rainbow.

The epidermis is the layer that bubbles up when we have a blister and as we know from this experience, it has no blood or nerves in it. The cells at the base of the epidermis continually divide and push the cells above them upwards. As these cells move up they die and become the dry flaky scales that fall off the skin surface. The cells in the epidermis die because a special protein called keratin is deposited in them. Keratin is an extremely important substance for it makes the skin waterproof. Without it land vertebrates like reptiles, birds and mammals would, like frogs, be able to survive only in damp places.

Skin Structures Made of Keratin

Claws, Nails and Hoofs

Reptiles, birds and mammals all have nails or claws on the ends of their toes. They protect the end of the toe and may be used for grasping, grooming, digging or in defense. They are continually worn away and grow continuously from a growth layer at their base (see diagram 5.1).

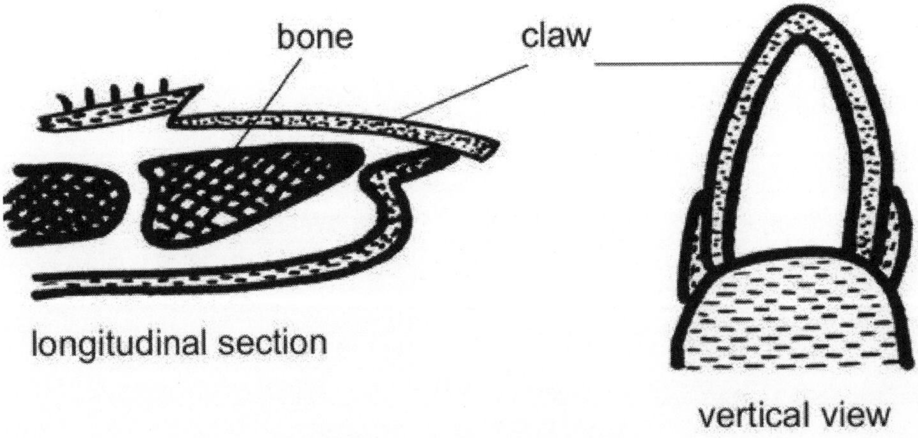

Fig. 5.1 A carnivore's claw

Hoofs are found in sheep, cows, horses etc. otherwise known as ungulate mammals . These are animals that have lost toes in the process of evolution and walk on the "nails" of the remaining toes. The hoof is a cylinder of horny material that surrounds and protects the tip of the toe.

Horns and Antlers

True horns are made of keratin and are found in sheep, goats and cattle. They are never branched and, once grown, are never shed. They consist of a core of bone arising in the dermis of the skin and are fused with the skull. The horn itself forms as a hollow cone-shaped sheath around the bone (see diagram 5.2).

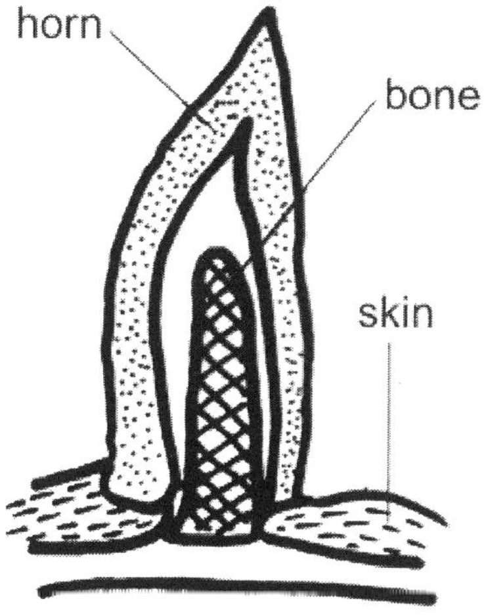

Fig. 5.2 - A horn

The antlers of male deer have quite a different structure. They are not formed in the epidermis and do not consist of keratin but are entirely of bone. They are shed each year and are often branched, especially in older animals. When growing they are covered in skin called velvet that forms the bone. Later the velvet is shed to leave the bony antler. The velvet is often removed artificially to be sold in Asia as a traditional medicine (see diagram 5.3).

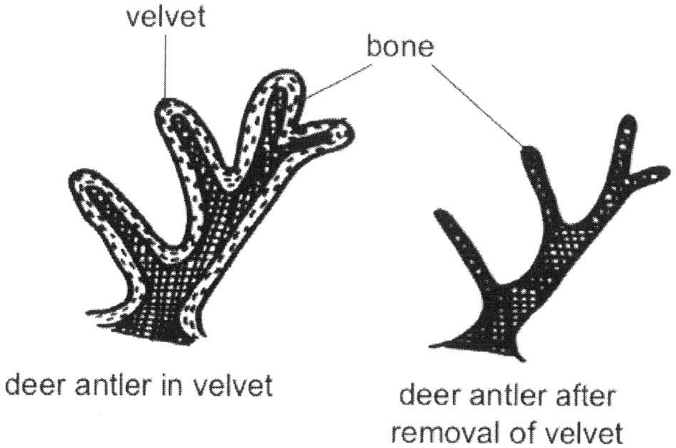

Fig. 5.3

Other animals have projections on their heads that are not true horns either. The horns on the head of giraffes are made of bone covered with skin and hair, and the 'horn' of a rhinoceros is made of modified and fused hair-like structures.

Hair

Hair is also made of keratin and develops in the epidermis. It covers the body of most mammals where it acts as an insulator and helps to regulate the temperature of the body (see below). The colour in hairs is formed from the same pigment, melanin that colours the skin. Coat colour may help camouflage animals and sometimes acts to attract the opposite sex.

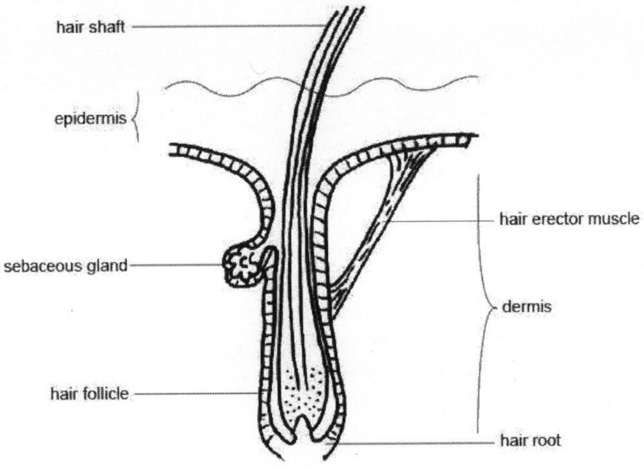

Fig. 5.4 A hair

Hairs lie in a follicle and grow from a root that is well supplied with blood vessels. The hair itself consists of layers of dead keratin - containing cells and usually lies at a slant in the skin. A small bundle of smooth muscle fibres (the hair erector muscle) is attached to the side of each hair and when this contracts the hair stands on end. This increases the insulating power of the coat and is also used by some animals to make them seem larger when confronted by a foe or a competitor.

The whiskers of cats and the spines of hedgehogs are examples of special types of hairs.

Feathers

The lightness and stiffness of keratin is also a key to bird flight. In the form of feathers it provides the large airfoils necessary for flapping and gliding flight. In another form, the light fluffy down feathers,also made of keratin, are some of the best natural insulators known. This superior insulation is necessary to help maintain the high body temperatures of birds.

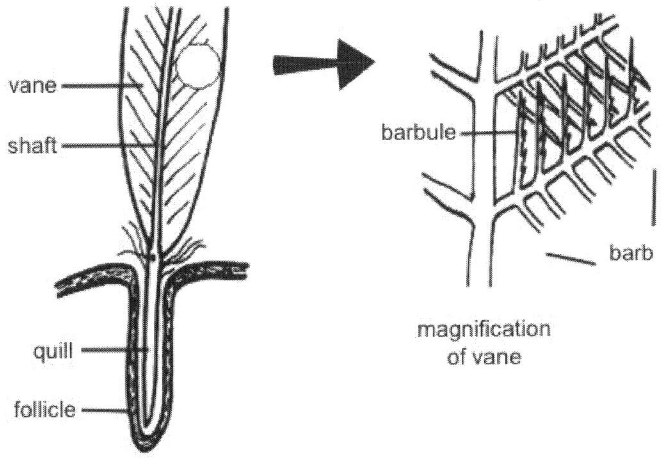

Fig. 5.5 A Contour Feather

Countour feathers are large feathers that cover the body, wings and tail. They have an expanded vane that provides the smooth, continuous surface that is required for effective flight. This surface is formed by barbs that extend out from the central shaft. If you look carefully at a feather you can see that on either side of each barb are thousands of barbules that lock together by a complex system of hooks and notches. if this arrangement becomes disrupted, the bird uses its beak to draw the barbs and barbules together again in an action known as preening.

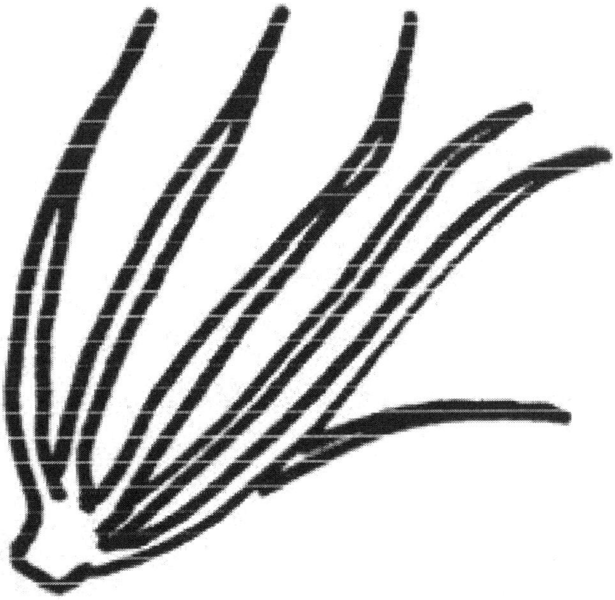

Fig. 5.6 A Down Feather

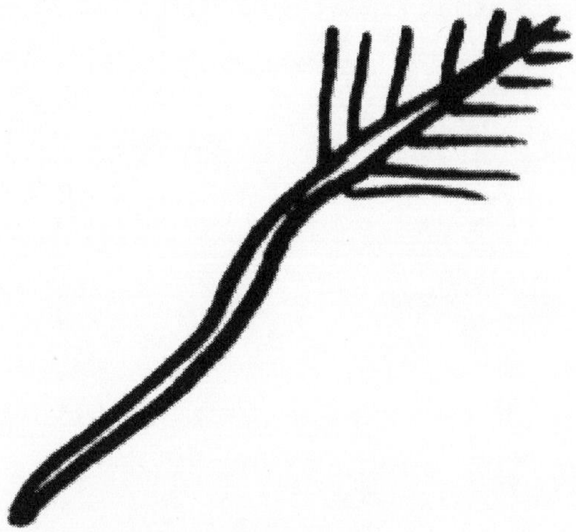

Fig. 5.7 A Pin Feather

Down feathers are the only feathers covering a chick and form the main insulation layer under the contour feathers of the adult. They have no shaft but consist of a spray of simple, slender branches (see diagram 5.6).

Pin feathers have a slender hair-like shaft often with a tiny tuft of barbs on the end. They are found between the other feathers and help tell a bird how its feathers are lying (see diagram 5.7).

Skin Glands

Glands are organs that produce and secrete fluids. They are usually divided into two groups depending upon whether or not they have channels or ducts to carry their products away. Glands with ducts are called exocrine glands and include the glands found in the skin as well as the glands that produce digestive enzymes in the gut. Endocrine glands have no ducts and release their products (hormones) directly into the blood stream. The pituitary and adrenal glands are examples of endocrine glands.

Most vertebrates have exocrine glands in the skin that produce a variety of secretions. The slime on the skin of fish and frogs is mucus produced by skin glands and some fish and frogs also produce poison from modified glands. In fact the skin glands of some frogs produce the most poisonous chemicals known. Reptiles and birds have a dry skin with few glands. The preen gland , situated near the base of the bird's tail, produces oil to help keep the feathers in good condition. Mammals have an array of different skin glands. These include the wax producing, sweat, sebaceous and mammary glands.

- Wax producing glands are found in the ears.
- Sebaceous glands secrete an oily secretion into the hair follicle. This secretion, known as

- sebum , keeps the hair supple and helps prevent the growth of bacteria.
- Sweat glands consist of a coiled tube and a duct leading onto the skin surface. Their appearance when examined under the microscope inspired one of the first scientists to observe them to call them "fairies' intestines". Sweat contains salt and waste products like urea and the evaporation of sweat on the skin surface is one of the major mechanisms for cooling the body of many mammals. Horses can sweat up to 30 litres of fluid a day during active exercise, but cats and dogs have few sweat glands and must cool themselves by panting. Scent in the sweat of many animals is used to mark territory or attract the opposite sex.

Mammary glands are only present in mammals. They are thought to be modified sebaceous glands and are present in both sexes but are rarely active in males (see diagram 5.8). The number of glands varies from species to species. They open to the surface in well-developed nipples. Milk contains proteins, sugars, fats and salts, although the exact composition varies from one species to another.

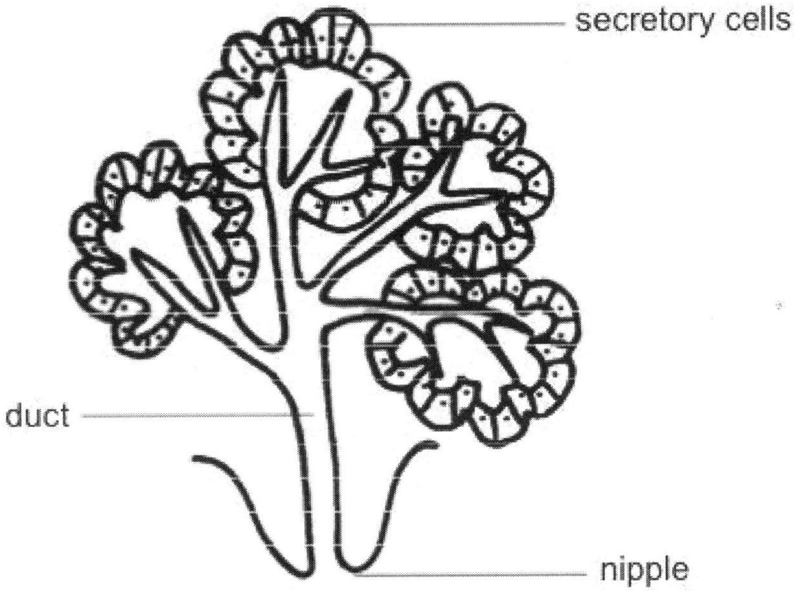

Fig. 5.8 A Mammary Gland

5.5 The Skin And Sun

A moderate amount of UV in sunlight is necessary for the skin to form vitamin D. This vitamin prevents bone disorders like rickets to which animals reared indoors are susceptible. Excessive exposure to the UV in sunlight can be damaging and the pigment melanin , deposited in cells at the base of the epidermis, helps to protect the underlying layers of the skin from this damage. Melanin also colours the skin and variations in the amount of melanin produces colours from pale yellow to black.

Sunburn And Skin Cancer

Excess exposure to the sun can cause sunburn. This is common in humans, but light skinned animals like cats and pigs can also be sunburned, especially on the ears. Skin cancer can also result from excessive exposure to the sun. As holes in the ozone layer increase exposure to the sun's UV rays, so too does the rate of skin cancer in humans and animals.

The Dermis

The underlying layer of the skin, known as the dermis, is much thicker but much more uniform in structure than the epidermis. It is composed of loose connective tissue with a felted mass of collagen and elastic fibres . It is this part of the skin of cattle and pigs etc. that becomes commercial leather when treated,. The dermis is well supplied with blood vessels, so cuts and burns that penetrate down into the dermis will bleed or cause serious fluid loss. There are also numerous nerve endings and touch receptors in the dermis because, of course, the skin is sensitive to touch, pain and temperature.

When looking at a section of the skin under the microscope you can see hair follicles, sweat and sebaceous glands dipping down into the dermis. However, these structures do not originate in the dermis but are derived from the epidermis.

In the lower levels of the dermis is a layer of fat or adipose tissue. This acts as an energy store and is an excellent insulator especially in mammals like whales with little hair.

The Skin And Temperature Regulation

Vertebrates can be divided into two groups depending on whether or not they control their internal temperature. Amphibia (frogs) and reptiles are said to be"cold blooded " (poikilothermic) because their body temperature approximately follows that of the environment. Birds and mammals are said to be warm blooded (homoiothermic) because they can maintain a roughly constant body temperature despite changes in the temperature of the environment.

Heat is produced by the biochemical reactions of the body (especially in the liver) and by muscle contraction. Most of the heat loss from the body occurs via the skin. It is therefore not surprising that many of the mechanisms for controlling the temperature of the body operate here.

Reduction Of Heat Loss

When an animal is in a cold environment and needs to reduce heat loss the erector muscles contract causing the hair or feathers to rise up and increase the layer of insulating air trapped by them.

Heat loss from the skin surface can also be reduced by the contraction of the abundant blood vessels that lie in the dermis. This takes blood flow to deeper levels, so reducing heat loss and causing pale skin.

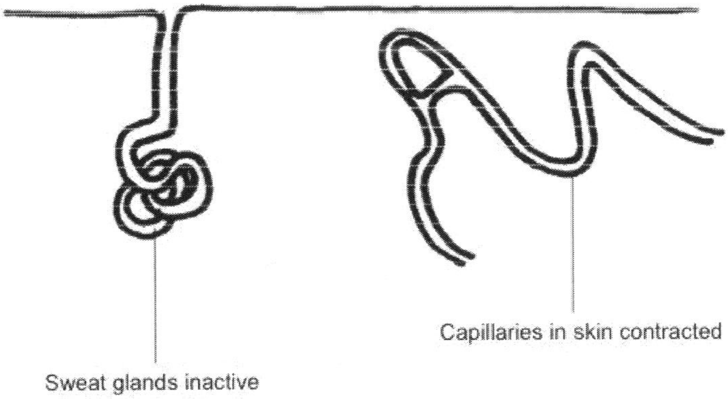

Fig. 5.9

Shivering caused by twitching muscles produces heat that also helps raise the body temper- ature.

Increase of Heat Loss

There are two main mechanisms used by animals to increase the amount of heat lost from the skin when they are in a hot environment or high levels of activity are increasing internal heat production. The first is the expansion of the blood vessels in the dermis so blood flows near the skin surface and heat loss to the environment can take place. The second is by the production of sweat from the sweat glands. The evaporation of this liquid on the skin surface produces a cooling effect.

The mechanisms for regulating body temperature are under the control of a small region of the brain called the hypothalamus . This acts like a thermostat.

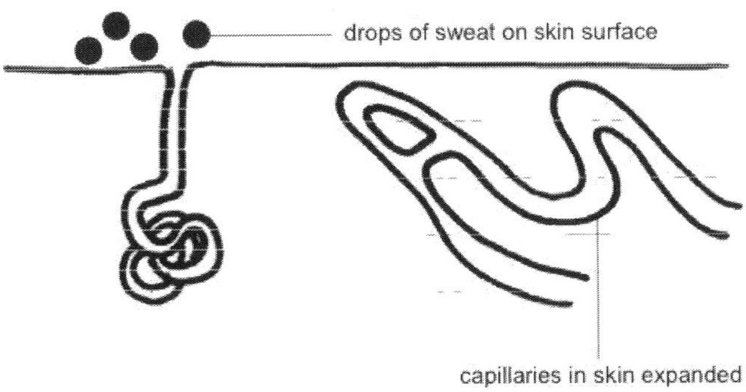

Fig. 5.10

Heat Loss And Body Size

The amount of heat that can be lost from the surface of the body is related to the area of skin an animal has in relation to the total volume of its body.

Small animals like mice have a very large skin area compared to their total volume. This means they tend to loose large amounts of heat and have difficulty keeping warm in cold weather. They may need to keep active just to maintain their body temperature or may hibernate to avoid the problem.

Large animals like elephants have the opposite problem. They have only a relatively small skin area in relation to their total volume and may have trouble keeping cool. This is one reason that these large animals tend to have sparse coverings of hair.

Summarys

- Skin consists of two layers: the thin epidermis and under it the thicker dermis.
- The Epidermis is formed by the division of base cells that push those above them towards the surface where they die and are shed.
- Keratin , a protein, is deposited in the epidermal cells. It makes skin waterproof.
- Various skin structures formed in the epidermis are made of keratin. These include: claws, nails, hoofs, horn, hair and feathers.
- Various Exocrine Glands (with ducts) formed in the epidermis include sweat, sebaceous, and mammary glands.

Worksheet

- Melanin deposited in cells at the base of the epidermis protects deeper cells from the harmful effects of the sun.
- The Dermis is composed of loose connective tissue and is well supplied with blood.
- Beneath the dermis is insulating adipose tissue .
- Body Temperature is controlled by: sweat, hair erection, dilation and contraction of dermal capillaries and shivering.

6

THE SKELETON

Objectives

After completing this section, you should know:

- the functions of the skeleton
- the basic structure of a vertebrae and the regions of the vertebral column

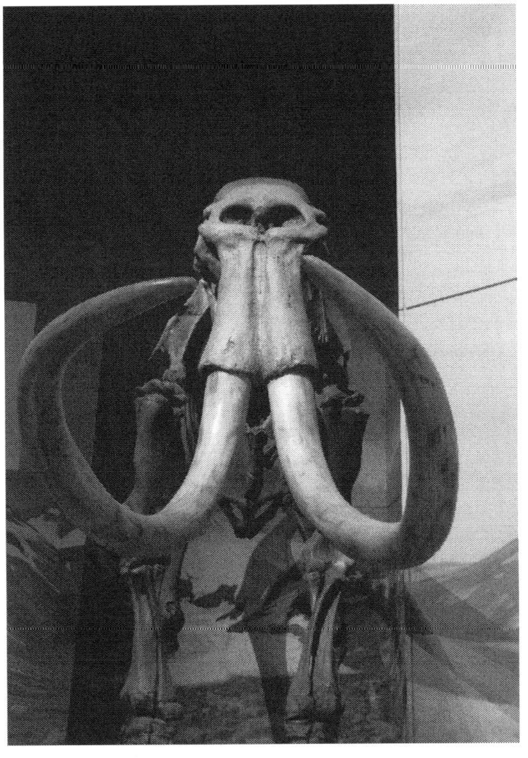

Fig. 6.1 original image by heschonga cc by

- the general structure of the skull

- the difference between 'true ribs' and 'floating ribs
- the main bones of the fore and hind limbs, and their girdles and be able to identify them in a live cat, dog, or rabbit

Fish, frogs, reptiles, birds and mammals are called vertebrates , a name that comes from the bony column of vertebrae (the spine) that supports the body and head. The rest of the skeleton of all these animals (except the fish) also has the same basic design with a skull that houses and protects the brain and sense organs and ribs that protect the heart and lungs and, in mammals, make breathing possible. Each of the four limbs is made to the same basic pattern. It is joined to the spine by means of a flat, broad bone called a girdle and consists of one long upper bone, two long lower bones, several smaller bones in the wrist or ankle and five digits.

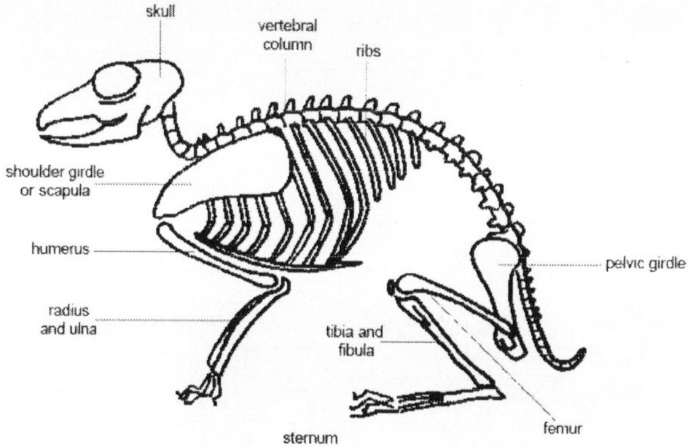

Fig. 6.2 The mammalian skeleton

The Vertebral Column

The vertebral column consists of a series of bones called vertebrae linked together to form a flexible column with the skull at one end and the tail at the other. Each vertebra consists of a ring of bone with spines (spinous process) protruding dorsally from it. The spinal cord passes through the hole in the middle and muscles attach to the spines making movement of the body possible.

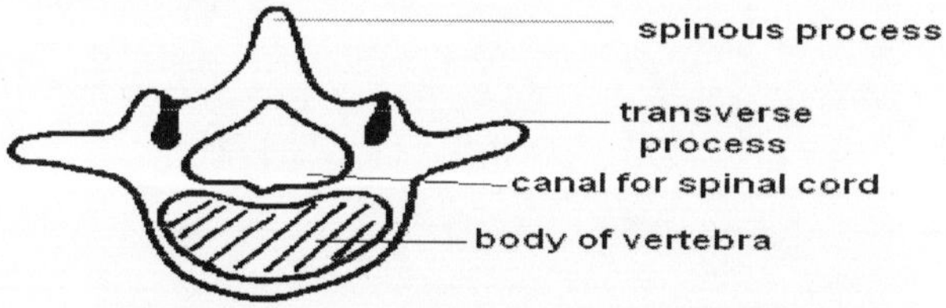

Fig. 6.3 Cross section of a lumbar vertebre

The shape and size of the vertebrae of mammals vary from the neck to the tail. In the neck there are cervical vertebrae with the two top ones, the atlas and axis , being specialised to support the head and allow it to nod "Yes" and shake "No". Thoracic vertebrae in the chest region have special surfaces against which the ribs move during breathing. Grazing animals like cows and giraffes that have to support weighty heads on long necks have extra large spines on their cervical and thoracic vertebrae for muscles to attach to. Lumbar vertebrae in the loin region are usually large strong vertebrae with prominent spines for the attachment of the large muscles of the lower back. The sacral vertebrae are usually fused into one solid bone called the sacrum that sits within the pelvic girdle . Finally there are a variable number of small bones in the tail called the coccygeal vertebrae.

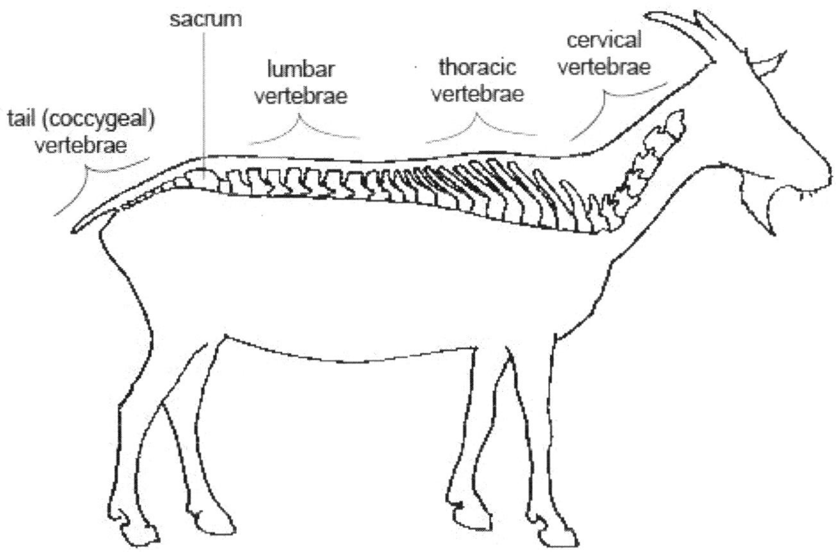

Fig. 6.4 The regions of the vertebral column dik

The Skull

The skull of mammals consists of 30 separate bones that grow together during development to form a solid case protecting the brain and sense organs. The "box "enclosing and pro- tecting the brain is called the cranium. The bony wall of the cranium encloses the middle and inner ears, protects the organs of smell in the nasal cavity and the eyes in sockets known as orbits . The teeth are inserted into the upper and lower jaws The lower jaw is known as the mandible. It forms a joint with the skull moved by strong muscles that allow an animal to chew. At the front of the skull is the nasal cavity, separated from the mouth by a plate of bone called the palate . Behind the nasal cavity and connecting with it are the sinuses . These are air spaces in the bones of the skull which help keep the skull as light as possible. At the base of the cranium is the foramen magnum , translated as "big hole", through which the spinal cord passes. On either side of this are two small, smooth rounded knobs or condyles that articulate (move against) the first or Atlas vertebra.

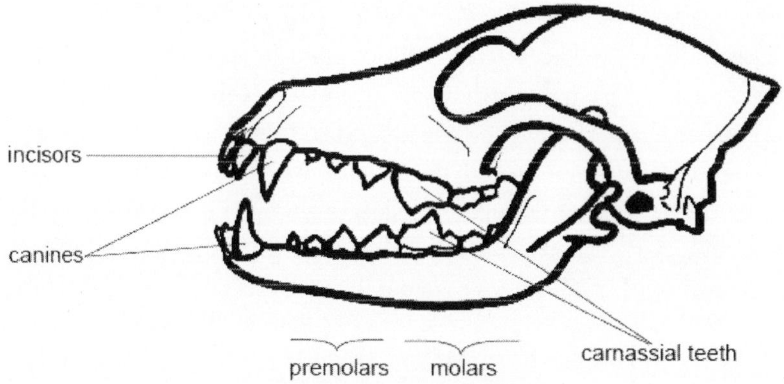

Fig. 6.5 A dog's skull

The Rib

Paired ribs are attached to each thoracic vertebra against which they move in breathing. Each rib is attached ventrally either to the sternum or to the rib in front by cartilage to form the rib cage that protects the heart and lungs. In dogs one pair of ribs is not attached ventrally at all. They are called floating ribs. Birds have a large expanded sternum called the keel to which the flight muscles (the 'breast" meat of a roast chicken) are attached.

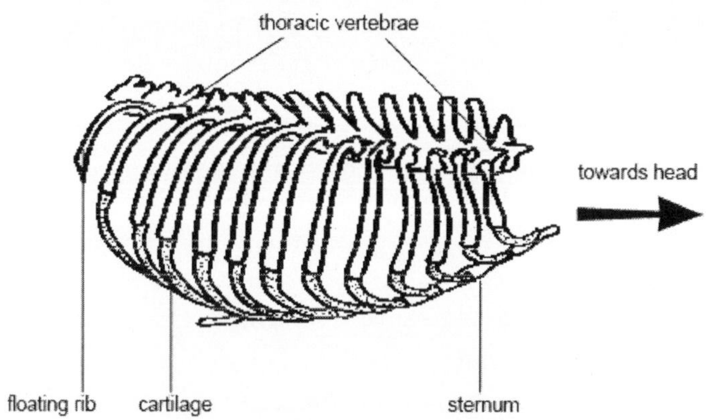

Fig. 6.6 The rib

The Forelimb

The forelimb consists of: Humerus, radius and ulna, carpals, metacarpals, digits or phalanges. The top of the humerus moves against (articulates with) the scapula at the shoulder joint. By changing the number, size and shape of the various bones, fore limbs have evolved to fit different ways of life. They have become wings for flying in birds and bats, flippers for swimming in whales, seals and porpoises, fast and efficient limbs for running in horses and arms and hands for holding and manipulating in primates).

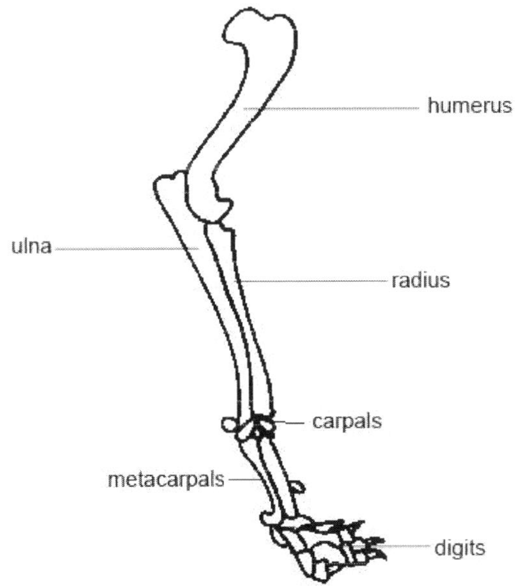

Fig. 6.7- Forelimb of a dog

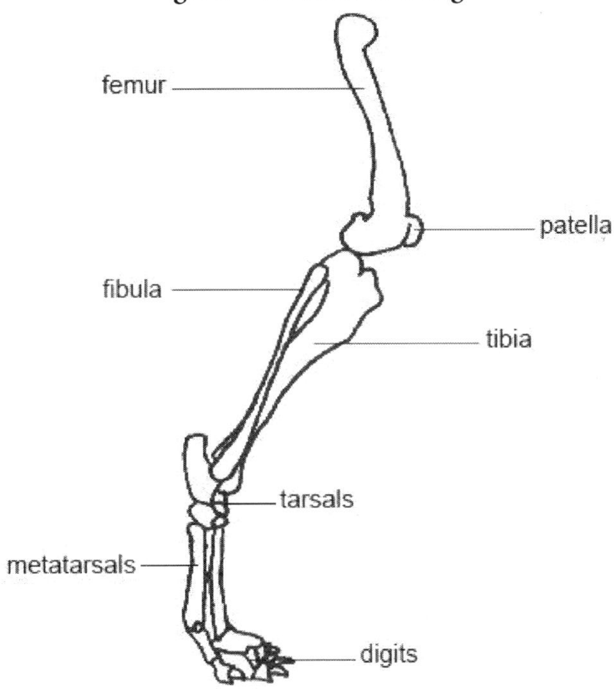

Fig. 6.8 Hindlimb of a dog

The Hind Limb

The hind limbs have a similar basic pattern to the forelimb. They consist of: femur, tibia and fibula, tarsals, metatarsals, digits or phalanges. The top of the femur moves against (articulates with) the pelvis at the hip joint.

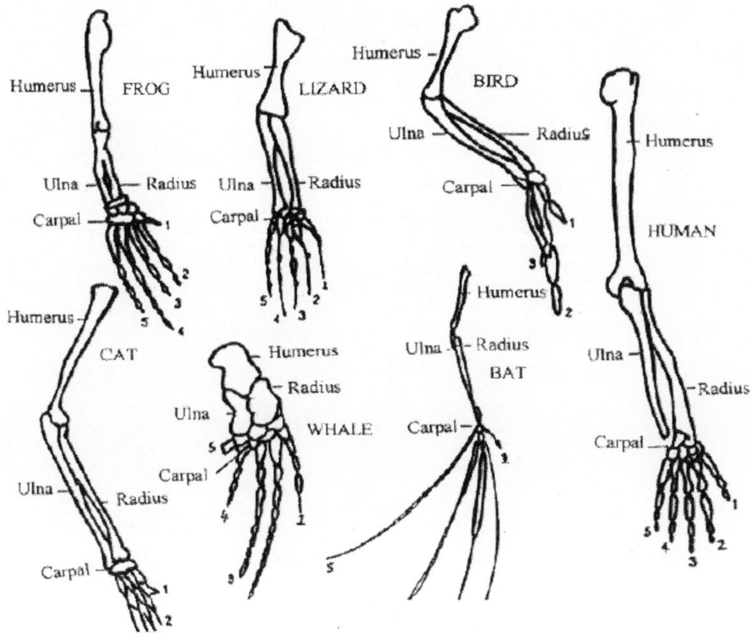

Fig. 6.9 Various vertebrate limbs

This diagram is wrong. The Long pastern or proximal phalanx is P1, not P3. The distal phalanx or coffin bone (called hoof there) is the 3rd phalanges. The patella or kneecap is embedded in a large tendon in front of the knee. It seems to smooth the movements of the knee. The legs of the horse are highly adapted to give it great galloping speed over long distances. The bones of the leg, wrist and foot are greatly elongated and the hooves are actually the tips of the third fingers and toes, the other digits having been lost or reduced (see diagram 6.9).

THE GIRDLES

The girdles pass on the "push" produced by the limbs to the body. The shoulder girdle or scapula is a triangle of bone surrounded by the muscles of the back but not connected directly to the spine. This arrangement helps it to cushion the body when landing after a leap and gives the forelimbs the flexibility to manipulate food or strike at prey. Animals that use their forelimbs for grasping, burrowing or climbing have a well-developed clavicle or collar bone. This connects the shoulder girdle to the sternum. Animals like sheep, horses and cows that use their forelimbs only for supporting the body and locomotion have no clavicle. The pelvic girdle or hipbone attaches the sacrum and the hind legs. It transmits the force of the leg-thrust in walking or jumping directly to the spine.

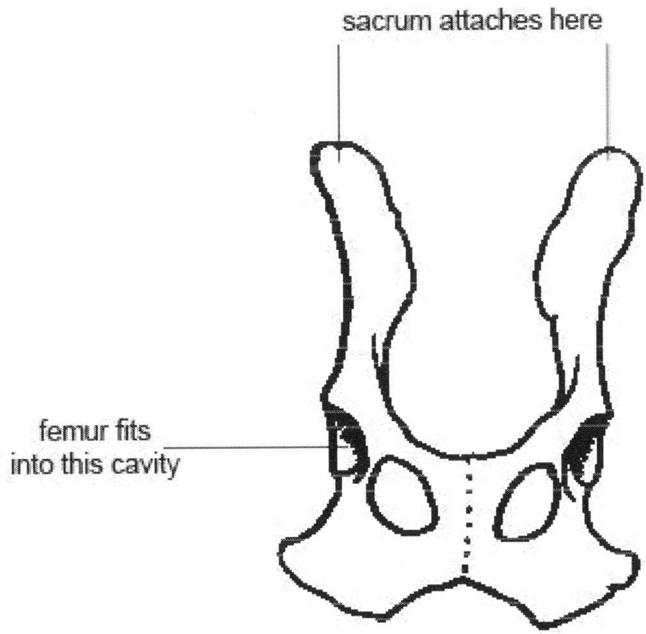

Fig. 6.10 The pelvic girdle

Categories Of Bones

People who study skeletons place the different bones of the skeleton into groups according to their shape or the way in which they develop. Thus we have long bones like the femur, radius and finger bones, short bones like the ones of the wrist and ankle, irregular bones

Bird Skeletons

like the vertebrae and flat bones like the shoulder blade and bones of the skull. Finally there are bones that develop in tissue separated from the main skeleton. These include sesamoid bones which include bones like the patella or kneecap that develop in tendons and visceral bones that develop in the soft tissue of the penis of the dog and the cow's heart.

Bird Skeletons

Although the skeleton of birds is made up of the same bones as that of mammals, many are highly adapted for flight. The most noticeable difference is that the bones of the forelimbs are elongated to act as wings. The large flight muscles make up as much as 1/5th of the body weight and are attached to an extension of the sternum called the keel . The vertebrae of the lower back are fused to provide the rigidity needed to produce flying movements. There are also many adaptations to reduce the weight of the skeleton. For instance birds have a beak rather than teeth and many of the bones are hollow.

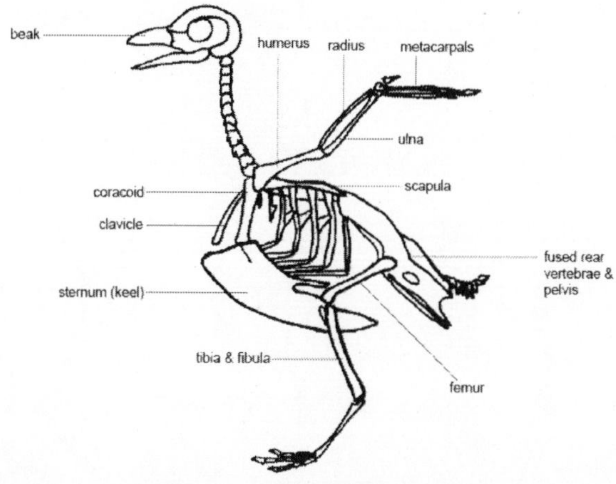

Fig. 6.11 - A bird's skeleton

THE STRUCTURE OF LONG BONES

A long bone consists of a central portion or shaft and two ends called epiphyses. Long bones move against or articulate with other bones at joints and their ends have flattened surfaces and rounded protuberances (condyles) to make this possible. If you carefully examine a long bone you may also see raised or rough surfaces. This is where the muscles that move the bones are attached. You will also see holes (a hole is called a foramen) in the bone. Blood vessels and nerves pass into the bone through these. You may also be able to see a fine line at each end of the bone. This is called the growth plate or epiphyseal line and marks the place where increase in length of the bone occurred.

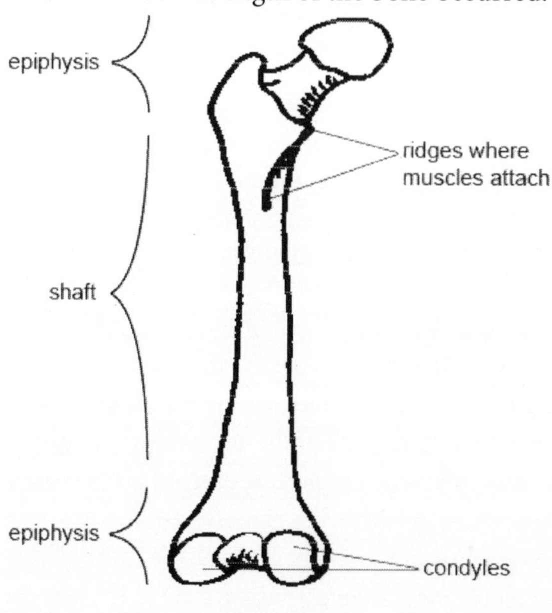

Fig. 6.12

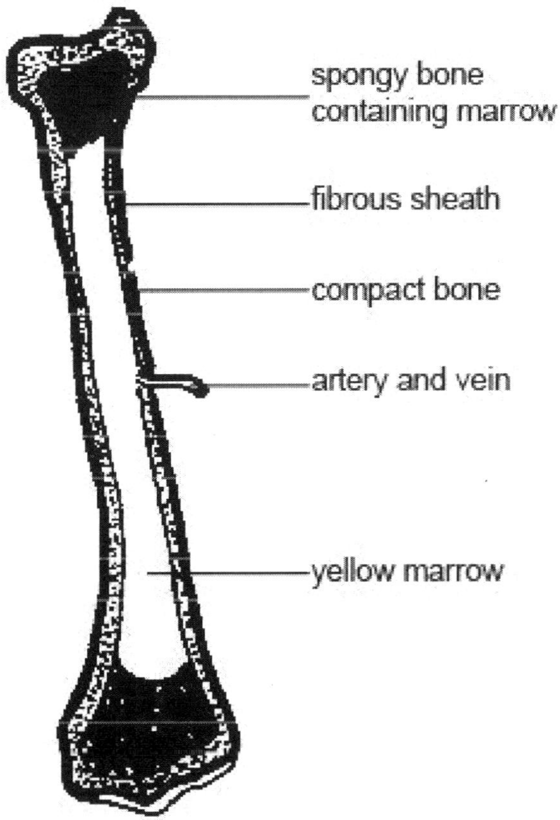

Fig. 6.13 - A longitudinal section through a long bone

If you cut a long bone lengthways you will see it consists of a hollow cylinder. The outer shell is covered by a tough fibrous sheath to which the tendons are attached. Under this is a layer of hard, dense compact bone. This gives the bone its strength. The central cavity contains fatty yellow marrow , an important energy store for the body, and the ends are made from honeycomb-like bony material called spongy bone. Spongy bone contains red marrow where red blood cells are made.

Compact Bone

Compact bone is not the lifeless material it may appear at first glance. It is a living dynamic tissue with blood vessels, nerves and living cells that continually rebuild and reshape the bone structure as a result of the stresses, bends and breaks it experiences. Compact bone is composed of microscopic hollow cylinders that run parallel to each other along the length of the bone. Each of these cylinders is called a Haversian system. Blood vessels and nerves run along the central canal of each Haversian system. Each system consists of concentric rings of bone material (the matrix) with minute spaces in it that hold the bone cells. The hard matrix contains crystals of calcium phosphate, calcium carbonate and magnesium salts with collagen fibres that make the bone stronger and somewhat flexible. Tiny canals connect the cells with each other and their blood supply.

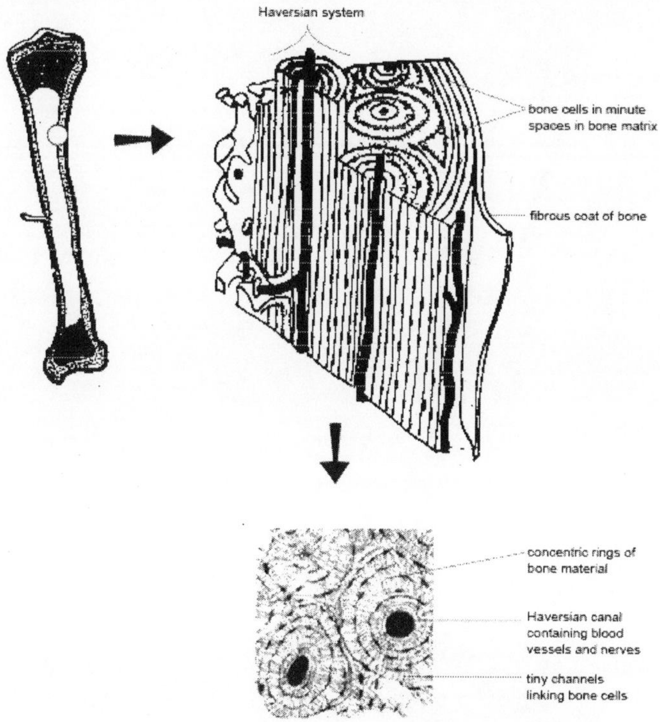

Fig. 6.14 Haversian systems of compact bone

SPONGY BONE

Spongy bone gives bones lightness with strength. It consists of an irregular lattice that looks just like an old fashioned loofah sponge. It is found on the ends of long bones and makes up most of the bone tissue of the limb girdles, ribs, sternum, vertebrae and skull. The spaces contain red marrow, which is where red blood cells are made and stored.

Bone Growth

The skeleton starts off in the foetus as either cartilage or fibrous connective tissue. Before birth and, sometimes for years after it, the cartilage is gradually replaced by bone. The long bones increase in length at the ends at an area known as the epiphyseal plate where new cartilage is laid down and then gradually converted to bone. When an animal is mature, bone growth ceases and the epiphyseal plate converts into a fine epiphyseal line.

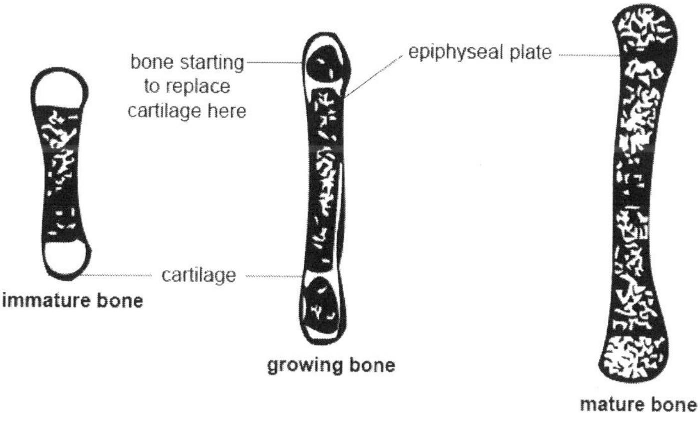

Fig. 6.15 A growing bone

Broken Bones

A fracture or break dramatically demonstrates the dynamic nature of bone. Soon after the break occurs blood pours into the site and cartilage is deposited. This starts to connect the broken ends together. Later spongy bone replaces the cartilage, which is itself replaced by compact bone. Partial healing to the point where some weight can be put on the bone can take place in 6 weeks but complete healing may take 3-4 months.

Joints

Joints are the structures in the skeleton where 2 or more bones meet. There are several different types of joints. Some are immovable once the animal has reached maturity. Examples of these are those between the bones of the skull and the midline joint of the pelvic girdle. Some are slightly moveable like the joints between the vertebrae but most joints allow free movement and have a typical structure with a fluid filled cavity separating the articulating surfaces (surfaces that move against each other) of the two bones. This kind of joint is called a synovial joint. The joint is held together by bundles of white fibrous tissue called ligaments and a fibrous capsule encloses the joint. The inner layers of this capsule secrete the synovial fluid that acts as a lubricant. The articulating surfaces of the bones are covered with cartilage that also reduces friction and some joints, e.g. the knee, have a pad of cartilage between the surfaces that articulate with each other.

The shape of the articulating bones in a joint and the arrangement of ligaments determine the kind of movement made by the joint. Some joints only allow a to and from gliding movement e.g. between the ankle and wrist bones; the joints at the elbow, knee and fingers are hinge joints and allow movement in two dimensions and the axis vertebra pivots on the atlas vertebra. Ball and socket joints , like those at the shoulder and hip, allow the greatest range of movement.

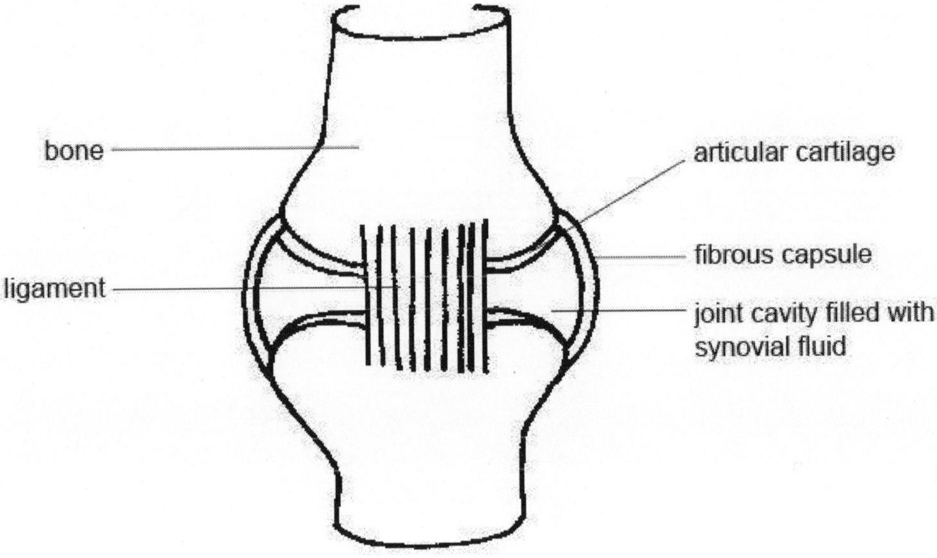

Fig. 6.16 - A synovial joint

Common Names of Joints

Some joints in animals are given common names that tend to be confusing. For example:

1. The joint between the femur and the tibia on the hind leg is our knee but the stifle

in animals.

2. Our ankle joint (between the tarsals and metatarsals) is the hock in animals
3. Our knuckle joint (between the metacarpals or metatarsals and the phalanges) is the

fetlock in the horse.

4. The "knee" on the horse is equivalent to our wrist (ie on the front limb between the radius and metacarpals).

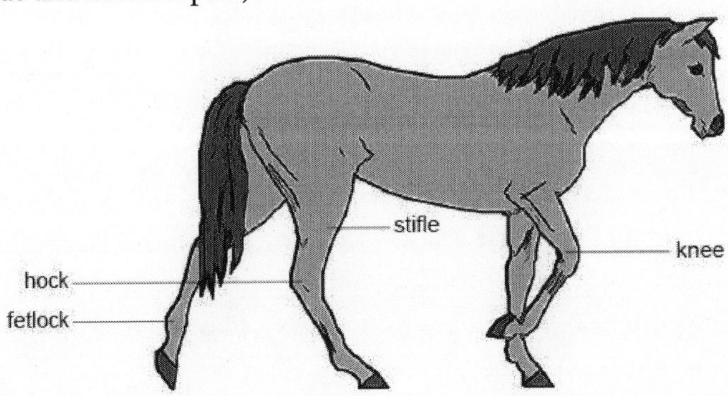

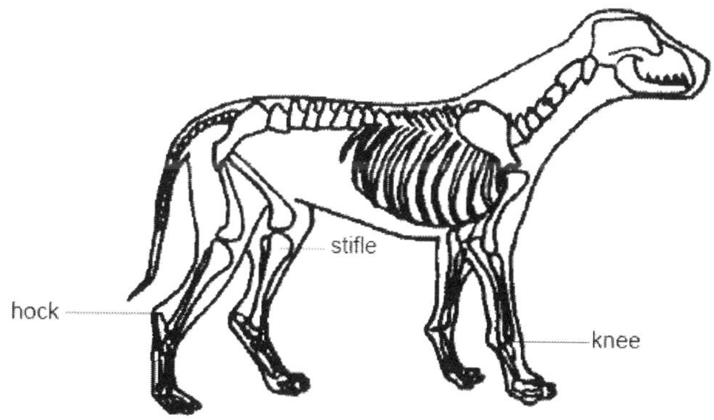

Fig. 6.17 b The names of common joints of a dog

LOCOMOTION

Different animals place different parts of the foot or forelimb on the ground when walking or running.

Humans and bears put the whole surface of the foot on the ground when they walk. This is known as plantigrade locomotion . Dogs and cats walk on their toes (digitigrade loco- motion) while horses and pigs walk on their "toenails" or hoofs. This is called unguligrade locomotion.

1. Plantigrade locomotion (on the "palms of the hand) as in humans and bears
2. Digitigrade locomotion (on the "fingers") as in cats and dogs
3. Unguligrade locomotion (on the "fingernails") as in horses

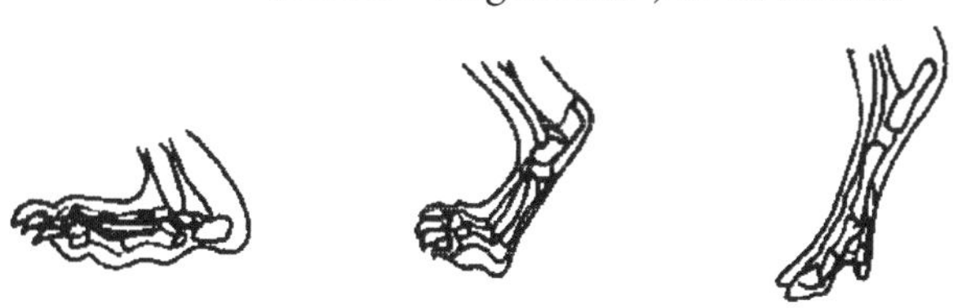

Fig. 6.18 Locomotion

Summary

- The skeleton maintains the shape of the body, protects internal organs and makes loco- motion possible.
- The vertebrae support the body and protect the spinal cord. They consist of: cervical vertebrae in the neck, thoracic vertebrae in the chest region which articulate with the ribs, lumbar vertebrae in the loin region, sacral vertebrae fused to the pelvis to form the sacrum and tail or coccygeal vertebrae .
- The skull protects the brain and sense organs. The cranium forms a solid box enclosing the brain. The mandible forms the jaw.

- The forelimb consists of the humerus, radius, ulna, carpals, metacarpals and phalanges . It moves against or articulates with the scapula at the shoulder joint.
- The hindlimb consists of the femur, patella, tibia, fibula, tarsals, metatarsals and digits.
- It moves against or articulates with the pelvis at the hip joint.
- Bones articulate against each other at joints .
- Compact bone in the shaft of long bones gives them their strength. Spongy bone at the ends reduces weight. Bone growth occurs at the growth plate .

Test Yourself

1. Name the bones which move against (articulate with)...

a) the humerus:

b) the thoracic vertebrae:

c) the pelvis:

2. Name the bones in the forelimb:

3. Where is the patella found?

4. Where are the following joints located?

a) The stifle joint:

b) The elbow joint:

c) The hock joint:

d) The hip joint:

5. Attach the following labels to the diagram of the long bone shown below.

a) compact bone

b) spongy bone

c) growth plate

d) fibrous sheath

e) (red marrow f) blood vessel

6. Attach the following labels to the diagram of a joint shown below

a) bone

b) articular cartilage

c) joint cavity

d) capsule

e) ligament

f) synovial fluid.

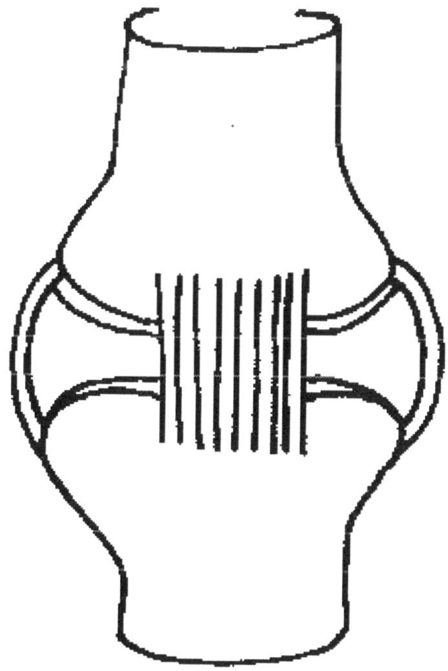

Fig. 6.19

7

MUSCLES

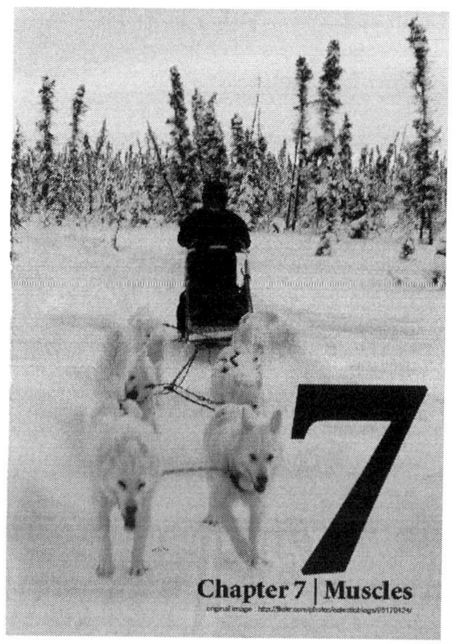

Fig. 7.1 original image by eclecticblogsa cc by

OBJECTIVES

After completing this section, you should know:

- The structure of smooth, cardiac and skeletal muscle and where they are found.
- What the insertion and origin of a muscle is.
- What flexion and extension of a muscle means.
- That muscles usually operate as antagonistic pairs.
- What tendons attach muscles to bones.

Muscles

Muscles make up the bulk of an animal's body and account for about half its weight. The meat on the chop or roast is muscle and is composed mainly of protein. The cells that make up muscle tissue are elongated and able to contract to a half or even a third of their length when at rest. There are three different kinds of muscle based on appearance and function: smooth, cardiac and skeletal muscle.

Types of Muscle

- Smooth muscle

Smooth or Involuntary muscle carries out the unconscious routine tasks of the body such as moving food down the digestive system, keeping the eyes in focus and adjusting the diameter of blood vessels. The individual cells are spindle-shaped, being fatter in the middle and tapering off towards the ends with a nucleus in the centre of the cell. They are usually found in sheets and are stimulated by the non-conscious or autonomic nervous system as well as by hormones.

- Cardiac muscle

Cardiac muscle is only found in the wall of the heart. It is composed of branching fibres that form a three-dimensional network. When examined under the microscope, a central nucleus and faint stripes or striations can be seen in the cells. Cardiac muscle cells contract spontaneously and rhythmically without outside stimulation, but the sinoatrial node (natural pacemaker) coordinates the heart beat. Nerves and hormones modify this rhythm.

- Skeletal muscle

Skeletal muscle is the muscle that is attached to and moves the skeleton, and is under voluntary control. It is composed of elongated cells or fibres lying parallel to each other. Each cell is unusual in that it has several nuclei and when examined under the microscope appears striped or striated. This appearance gives the muscle its names of striped or striated muscle. Each cell of striated muscle contains hundreds, or even thousands, of microscopic fibres each one with its own striped appearance. The stripes are formed by two different sorts of protein that slide over each other making the cell contract.

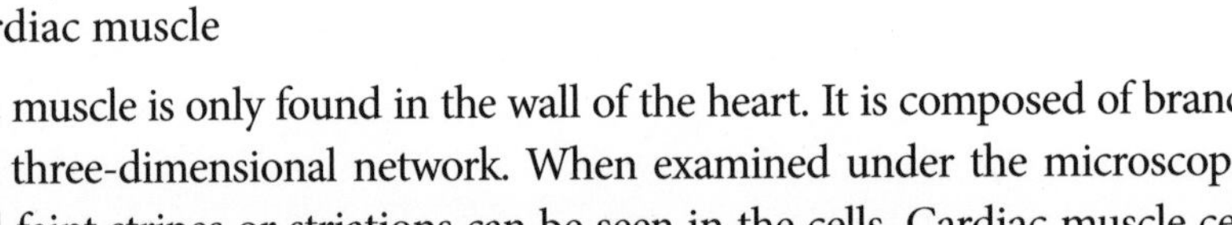

Fig. 7.2 - A striped muscle cell

MUSCLE CONTRACTION

Muscle contraction requires energy and muscle cells have numerous mitochondria. However, only about 15% of the energy released by the mitochondria is used to fuel muscle contraction. The rest is released as heat. This is why exercise increases body temperature and makes animals sweat or pant to rid themselves of this heat.

What we refer to as a muscle is made up of groups of muscle fibres surrounded by connective tissue. The connective tissue sheaths join together at the ends of the muscle to form tough white bands of fibre called tendons . These attach the muscles to the bones. Tendons are similar in structure to the ligaments that attach bones together across a joint.

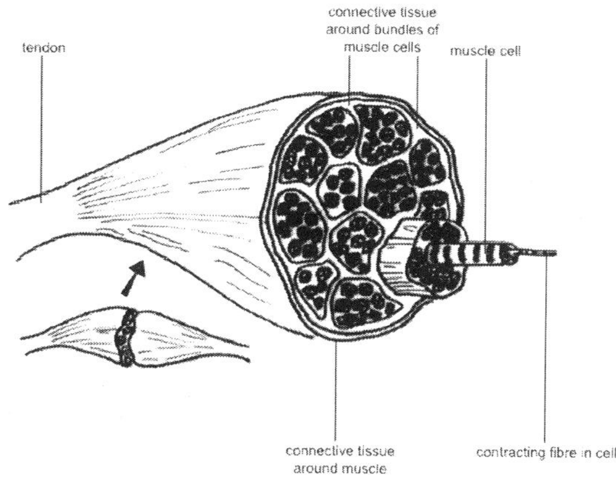

Fig. 7.3 The structure of a muscle Remember:

Tendons Tie muscles to bones and

Ligaments Link bones at joints

Structure of a muscle

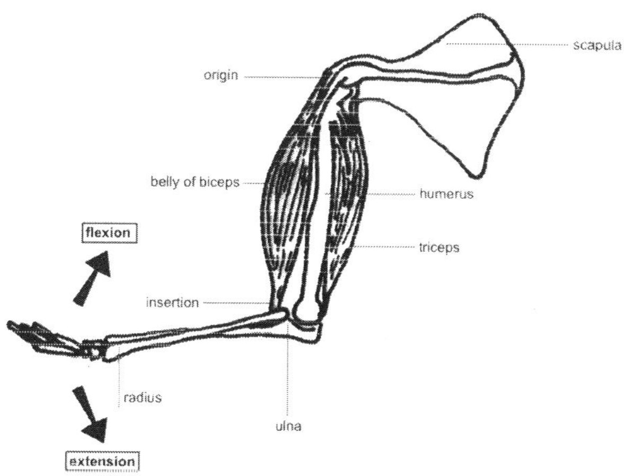

Fig. 7.4

A single muscle is fat in the middle and tapers towards the ends. The middle part, which gets fatter when the muscle contracts, is called the belly of the muscle. If you contract your biceps muscle in your upper arm you may feel it getting fatter in the middle. You may also notice that the biceps is attached at its top end to bones in your shoulder while at the bottom it is attached to bones in your lower arm. Notice that the bones at only one end move when you contract the biceps. This end of the muscle is called the insertion. The other end of the muscle, the origin , is attached to the bone that moves the least.

Antagonistic muscles

Skeletal muscles usually work in pairs. When one contracts the other relaxes and vice versa. Pairs of muscles that work like this are called antagonistic muscles . For example the muscles in the upper forearm are the biceps and triceps. Together they bend the elbow. When the biceps contracts (and the triceps relaxes) the lower forearm is raised and the angle of the joint is reduced. This kind of movement is called flexion . When the triceps is contracted (and the biceps relaxes), the angle of the elbow increases. The term for this movement is extension .

When you or animals contract skeletal muscle it is a voluntary action. For example, you make a conscious decision to walk across the room, raise the spoon to your mouth or smile. There is however, another way in which contraction of muscles attached to the skeleton happens that is not under voluntary control. This is during a reflex action , such as jerking your hand away from the hot stove you have touched by accident.

SUMMARY

- There are three different kinds of muscle tissue: smooth muscle in the walls of the gut and blood

vessels; cardiac muscle in the heart and skeletal muscle attached to the skeleton.

- Tendons attach skeletal muscles to the skeleton.
- Ligaments link bones together at a joint.
- Skeletal muscles work in pairs known as antagonistic pairs. As one contracts the other in the

pair relaxes.

- Flexion is the movement that reduces the angle of a joint. Extension increases the angle

of a joint.

Test Yourself

1. ***What kind of muscle tissue:***

a) moves bones:

b) makes the heart pump blood:

c) pushes food along the intestine:

d) makes your mouth form a smile:

e) makes the hair stand up when cold:

f) makes the diaphragm contract for breathing in:

2. What structure connects a muscle to a bone?
3. What is the insertion of a muscle?
4. Which muscle is antagonistic to the biceps?
5. Name 3 other antagonistic pairs and tell what they do.
6. When you bend your knee what movement are you making?
7. When you straighten your ankle joint what movement happens?
8. What organelles provide the energy that muscles need?
9. State the difference between a tendon and a ligament.
10. In the section "Skeletal Muscle" there are 2 proteins mentioned. Name these proteins, state their size difference, and tell what they actually do to help produce movement.

8

CARDIOVASCULAR SYSTEM

The cardiovascular system comprises the heart, veins, arteries, and capillary beds. The atrioventricular (mitral and tricuspid) and semilunar (aortic and pulmonic) valves keep blood flowing in one direction through the heart, and valves in large veins keep blood flowing back toward the heart. The rate and force of contraction of the heart and the degree of constriction or dilatation of blood vessels are determined by the autonomic nervous system (sympathetic and parasympathetic) and hormones produced either by the heart and blood vessels (ie, paracrine or autocrine) or at a distance from the heart and blood vessels (ie, endocrine).

The circulatory system consists of the cardiovascular system and lymphatic system. Cardiovascular system conducts blood and is composed of arteries, veins, capillary nets, and the heart. Lymphatic system is constituted by more heterogeneous structures like lymphatic vessels, lymphatic ganglia, nodules, and by organs like spleen and thymus.

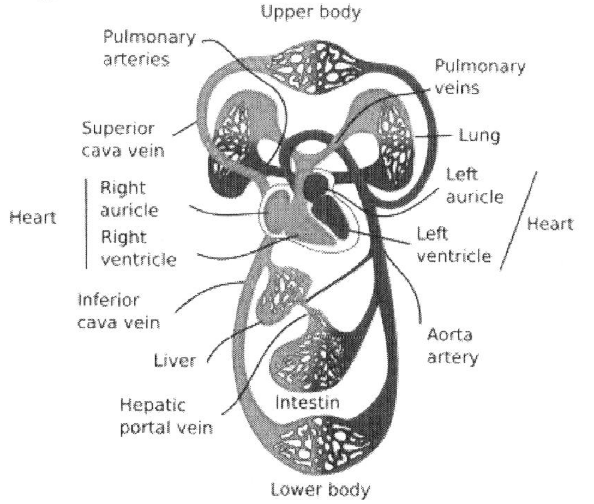

Fig. 8.1 Cardiovascular system in mammals.

The cardiovascular system is the main system for communication between different parts of the body of animals. It pumps and conducts the blood to irrigate the every part of the body. Blood is necessary for transporting food, waste products, oxygen, carbon dioxide, hormones and immune system cells. It also has other functions like keeping a constant body temperature.

The cardiovascular system is a double circuit, one irrigating the lungs, and the other irrigating the rest of the body. Both start and end in the heart, which is the organ in charge of keeping the blood in permanent motion. The pattern of blood vessels is the same in the two circuits: heart, arteries, arterioles, capillary net, small veins, veins and heart again. Sometimes, arterioles or small veins may be found connecting two capillary nets. This is a portal system, like the hepatic portal system that include the intestine and liver.

Arteries and veins are made up of three layers or tunics: tunica intima, tunica media and tunica adventitia. The tunica intima is the internal one, in contact with the blood, and it is constituted of a squamous simple epithelium (endothelium), a basal lamina, and a layer of loose connective tissue. The tunica media is mainly composed of smooth muscle cells. The tunica adventitia is the most external one and is connective tissue. Arteries and arterioles show thicker walls that veins and small veins, respectively, to resist stronger blood pressures because they are closer to the heart. Arteries usually have smaller diameter that veins that, together with their thicker walls, make them more rounded in histological sections, whereas veins show more irregular shapes.

Arteries and large veins contain other small blood vessels irrigating their walls, which are known as " vasa vasorum" (vessels of the vessels). This net of internal vessels is located closer to the tunica adventitia in arteries and closer to the lumen in veins. Arteries are more easily damaged that veins during pathological processes because the part of the tunica media (is mostly smooth muscle) close to the lumen is less irrigated. In the wall of arteries and veins there are nerve endings that modulate de contraction strength of the smooth muscle.

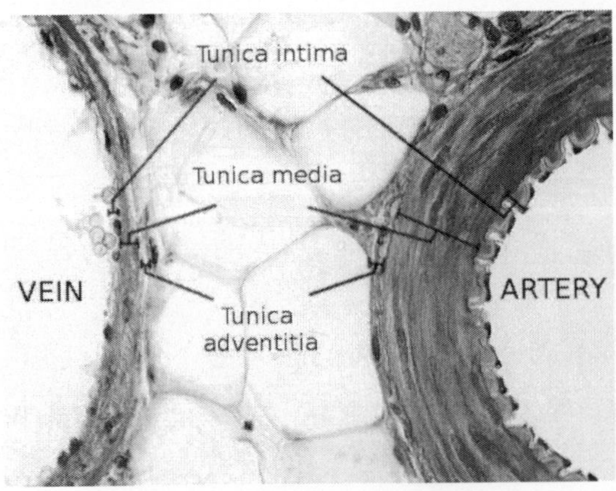

Fig. 8.2

Layers or tunics in a vein (on the left) and in an artery (on the right). Both are medium size vessels. Note the different thickness of the tunica media between the two vessels.

Arteries

Arteries are vessels conducting the blood in the heart-organ direction. The walls of arteries are thick to withstand the blood pressured produced by heart beating. According to the diameter, arteries are usually classified in large or elastic, medium or muscle and small or arterioles.

Elastic artery

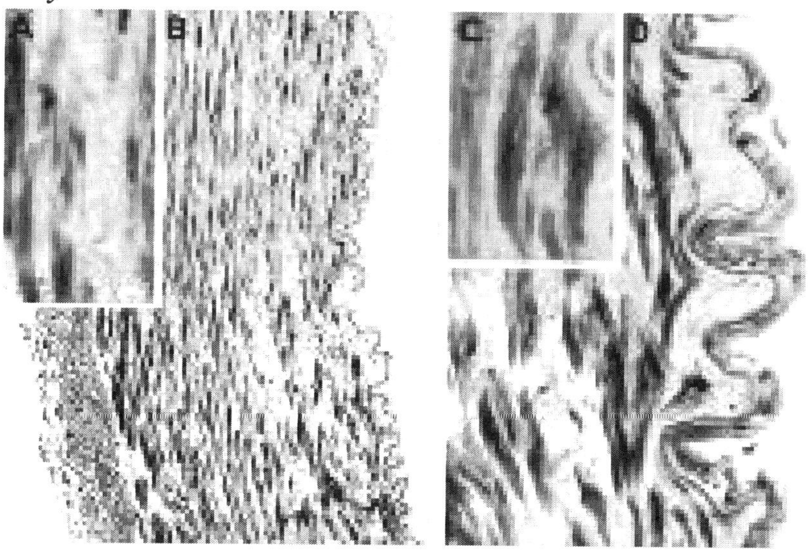

Fig. 8.3

Elastic artery.

Blood leaves the heart by the aorta and pulmonary arteries. Both get branched near the heart. These arteries and their first branches are regarded as elastic arteries. Their walls contain a large amount of the elastic fibers that make them recover a normal diameter after an enlargement produced by a heart beat. Elastic arteries show a thick tunica intima. The endothelium is made up of cells having tight junctions and desmosomes that keep cells well attached to each other. The major axis of the cells is oriented parallel to the direction of the blood flux. Subendothelial layer is connective tissue with collagen and elastic fibers, and some smooth muscle cells. The elastic lamina, which separates tunica intima from tunica media, is thin and sometime difficult to be observed. The tunica media is very thick, mostly made up of elastic and collagen fibers and many smooth muscle cells. The tunica adventitia es a layer of connective tissue with fibroblasts. Here there are not smooth muscle fibers. It is of notice that smooth muscle fibers of elastic arteries, besides of being responsible for the artery diameter by cell contraction, synthesize and release elastic and collagen fibers, i.e. they take the role of producing extracellular matrix.

Muscular arteries

Muscular arteries are medium size arteries, with varible diameters, and their histological organization is a transition between the elastic arteries and arterioles. The size of muscular arteries ranges from 0,1 to 10 mm in diameter. So that larger muscular arteries are more similar to elastic arteries and the smaller ones are more like arterioles. Proportionally, they contain less elastic fibers and more smooth muscle cells than elastic arteries.

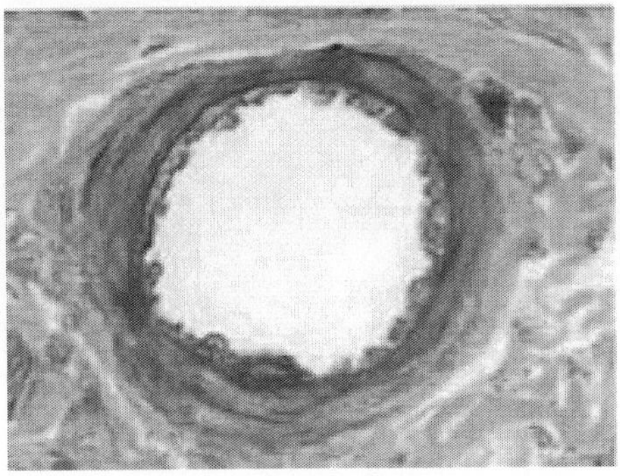

Fig. 8.4

ARTERIOLES.

Small arteries and arterioles

The diameter of small arteries and arterioles is variable, and they are identified by the number of layers of smooth muscle cells. As a consensus, small arteries show from 2 to 8 layers of smooth muscle. Arterioles have 1 to 2 layers and their diameter is about 30 μm. Arterioles are the main responsible for controlling the flow of blood that enters the capillary net by contracting their smooth muscle cells. Actually, these muscle cells are usually slightly contracted so they can regulate precisely the stream of blood. Both small arteries and arterioles have the same three tunics that are found in other arteries.

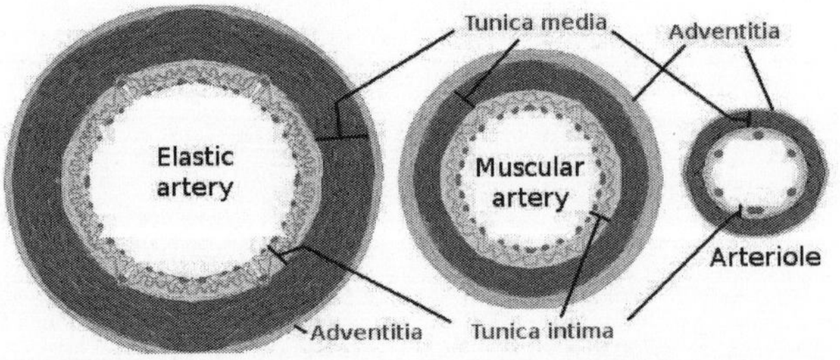

Fig. 8.5 Tunicae in the arteries with different diameters

Capillaries

Capillaries are the smallest blood vessels, sometimes even smaller than a red blood cell. The interchange of gases and substances between blood and tissues occurs mainly through the capillary endothelium. Capillary walls are made up by the endothelium and a basal lamina, and lack any other layer, so that the gases and substances interchange is facilitated. Capillaries are organized in widely distributed nets that irrigated all the organs of the body. This type or irrigation is known as perfusion.

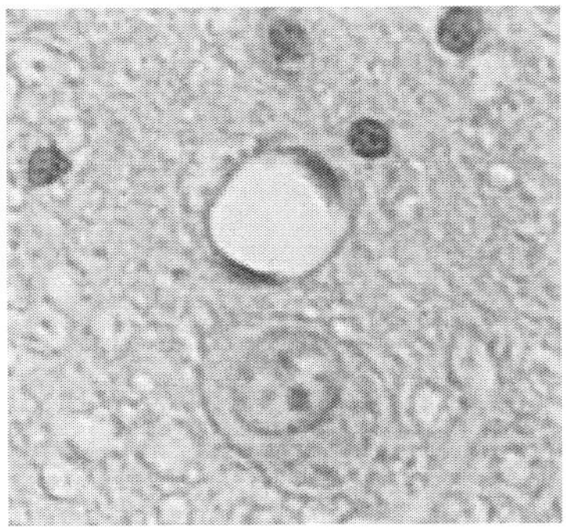

Fig. 8.6 Capillaries.

Endothelium can be continuous, fenestrated and discontinuous according to their cellular features and organization. Continuous endothelium is the more abundant capillary type. The endothelial cells seal the intercellular spaces so tightly that only the smallest molecules can cross the endothelium through the intercellular spaces. These endothelial cells show many cytoplasmic vesicles that indicate strong endocytocis and exocytosis processes. Fenestrated endothelium shows endothelial cells with channels or passages that connect directly blood with basal lamina and inner tissues. They are frequent in endocrine glands and intestine, places where the flux of substances to the blood is very intense. Discontinuous or sinusoidal endothelium is less frequent. Its endothelial cells do not completely seal the intercelular spaces, so that substances and even cells can cross freely the endothelium. It is found in the liver, bone marrow and spleen.

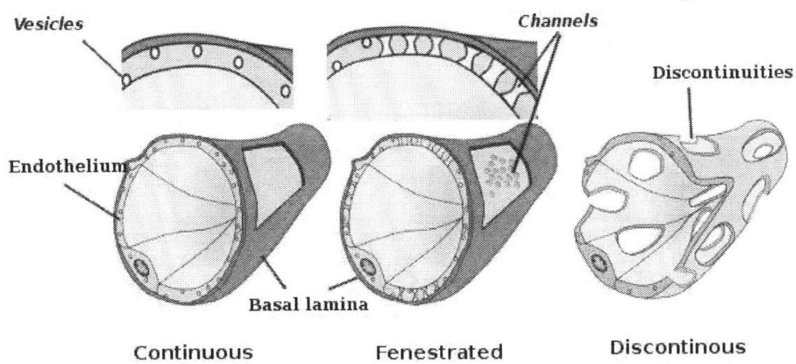

Fig. 8.7 Three types of capillaries.

Veins

Veins show the same structural organization as arteries. However, veins usually have larger diameters and the tunica media is not so well-developed. In addition, many veins, particularly those in the limbs, contain valves in the lumen preventing blood going in the wrong direction, that may be caused by gravity or by mechanical pressures. Veins are classified according to their size: large, medium, and small veins or venules.

Large veins

Large veins have a diameter of about 10 mm. Their tunica intima is formed of endothelium, scarce subendothelial tissue and few smooth muscle cells. The differences between tunica intima and tunica media are not easyly distinguished. The tunica media is thin with smooth muscle fibers perpendicularly arranged to the long axis of the vessel. The tunica adventitia, the thicker layer of the large veins, is made up of connective tissue and muscle fibers longitudinally arranged.

Middle-sized veins

These veins are smaller (about 10 mm in diameter) than larger veins and account for most of the veins of the organism. The shape of the medium-sized veins is more irregular that arteries and the three tunicae can be observed. The tunica intima shows endothelium, basal lamina and a thin layer of connective tissue containing some smooth muscle cells. Sometimes, an internal elastic membrane can be distinguished. The tunica media, although thinner than in the larger arteries, show several layers of smooth muscle cells scattered among connective tissue. The tunica adventitia, which is formed by connective tissue, is thicker than the tunica media.

Venules

There are two types of venules: postcapillary and muscular. Postcapillary veins receive the blood directly from capillaries. They have a very small diameter (about 0,1 mm). Influenced by molecular signals, the adhesion properties of the endothelial cells change frequently, which allow linphocytes and blood serum to easily cross the endothelial layer. These venules do not show a "true" tunica media. Muscular venules, about 1 mm in diameter, are located after the poscapillary venules. They have a tunica media with one or two layers of smooth muscle cells. They also show a thin tunica adventitia.

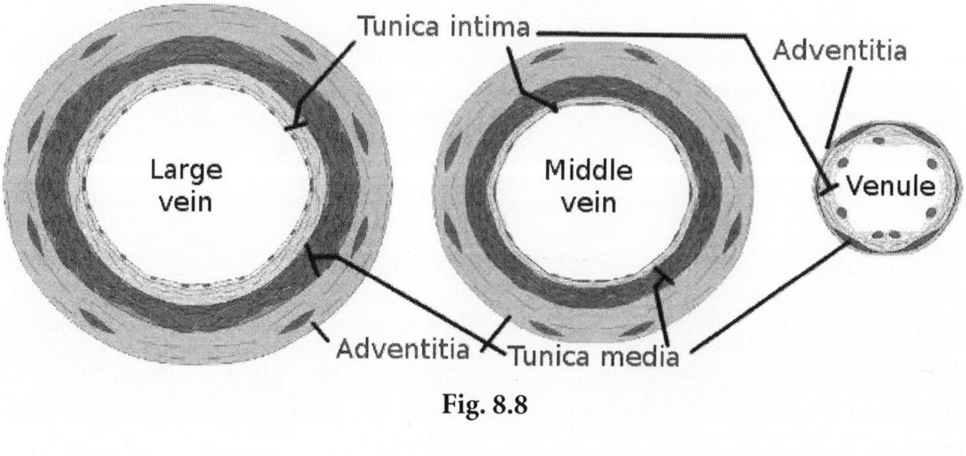

Fig. 8.8

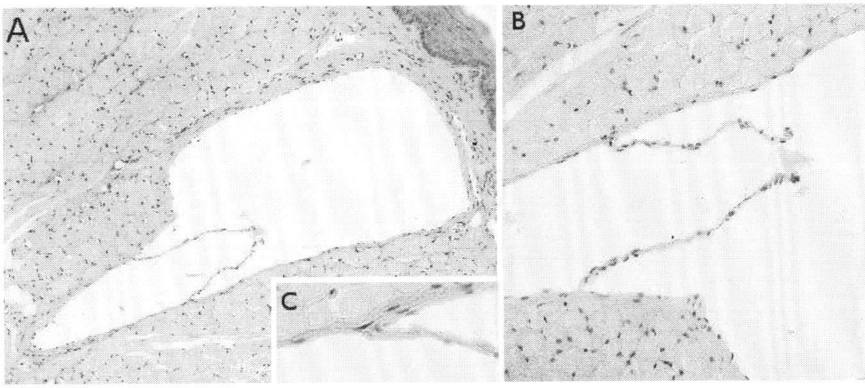

Fig. 8.9

Organization of vein tunicae in veins with different diameter. Vein valves are not depicted. Image showing a vein valve located in the transition between two veins of different diameter. B and C images are details of image A. The direction of the blood flow is from the left toward the right.

Heart

The heart is the organ that pumps the blood through the circulatory system, helped by the body movement. It is mostly made up of cardiac muscle cells, which are found only in this organ.

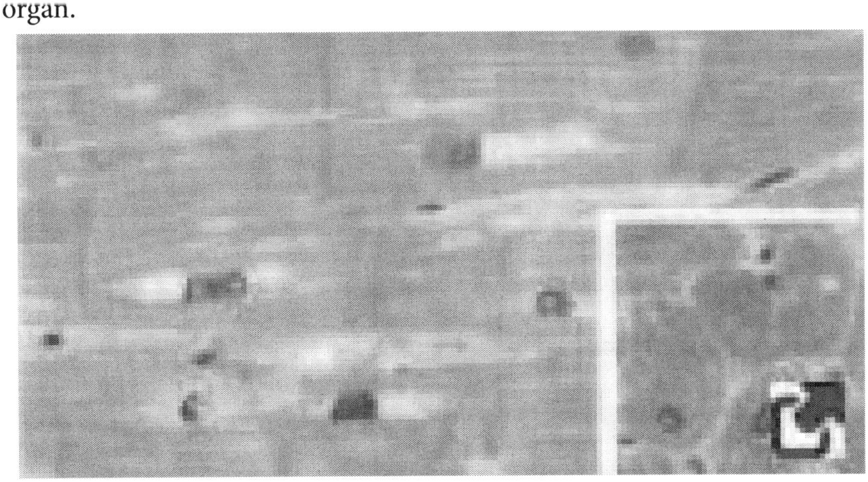

Fig. 8.10

Cardiac muscle.

The mammal heart has four chambers, two ventricles to pump the blood, and two auricles, one that gathers the pulmonary blood and the other collects the blood from the rest of the body. The two auricles are separated by the interventricular septum and the two ventricles by the ventricular septum. In each of the auricle entrances there is a valve that prevent the blood reflux.

The walls of the ventricles and auricles are made up of three layers: epicardium, myocardium and endocardium. The epicardium is the outer layer composed of mesothelium outward and connective tissue inward. Blood vessels and nerves that enter the cardiac muscle run through the epicardium. Many adipose cells are also found in this layer. Myocardium is mostly cardiac muscular cells, intermingled with scarce connective tissue. In ventricles, the myocardium is thicker than in the auricles, and shows an inner and an outer layers. The muscles of the outer layer are arranged in spirals and swirls, whereas the inner wrap around the ventricles and auricles. The endocardium is formed of an endothelium, in contact with the blood, and connective tissue containing some smooth muscle cells. Connective tissue in the endocardium, in contact with the myocardium, contains blood vessels and nerves.

The interventricular septum (or ventricular septum) is composed of cardiac muscle lined by endothelium. The interauricular septum (or atrial septum) is thinner and show the same tisular organization and the interventricular septum, although it is a fibrous structure in some parts.

Cardiac valves are connective tissue cavered by endothelium. From the inner to the outer part, each valve is made up of three layers: fibrosa, spongiosa and ventricularis. They contain different types of connective tissue: dense, loose and dense, respectively.

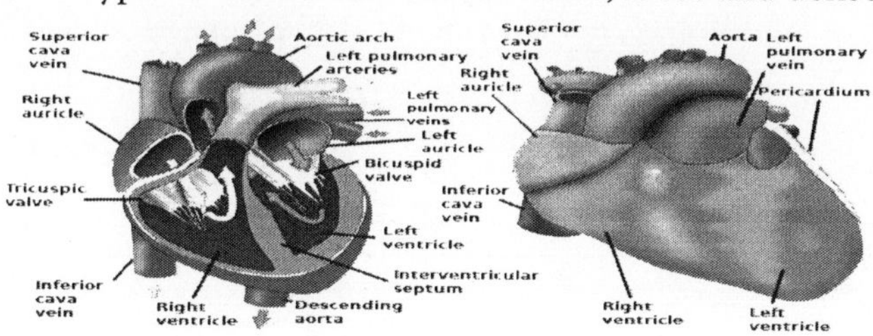

Fig. 8. 10 Main components of the mammalian heart.

CIRCULATORY SYSTEM ARCHITECTURE

The circulatory system is effectively a network of cylindrical vessels: the arteries, veins, and capillaries that emanate from a pump, the heart. In all vertebrate organisms, as well as some invertebrates, this is a closed-loop system, in which the blood is not free in a cavity. In a closed circulatory system, blood is contained inside blood vessels and circulates unidirectionally from the heart around the systemic circulatory route, then returns to the heart again.

As opposed to a closed system, arthropods– including insects, crustaceans, and most mollusks– have an 'open' circulatory system. In an open circulatory system, the blood is not enclosed in blood vessels but is pumped into an open cavity called a hemocoel and is called hemolymph because the blood mixes with the interstitial fluid. As the heart beats and the animal moves, the hemolymph circulates around the organs within the body cavity and then reenters the hearts through openings called ostia. This movement allows for nutrient exchange, and in some organisms lacking direct gas exchange sites, a basic mechanism to transport gasses beyond the exchange site. Because the gas exchange in many open-circulatory systems tends to be relatively low for metabolically-active organs and tissues, a tradeoff exists between this system and the much more energy-consuming, harder-to-maintain closed system.

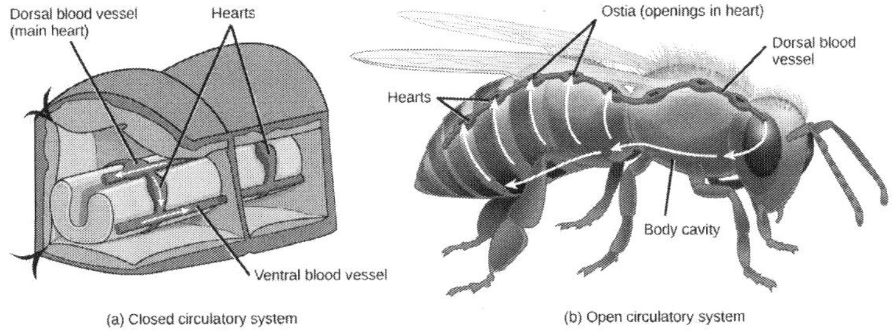

Fig. 8.11

In (a) closed circulatory systems, the heart pumps blood through vessels that are separate from the interstitial fluid of the body. Most vertebrates and some invertebrates, like this annelid earthworm, have a closed circulatory system. In (b) open circulatory systems, a fluid called hemolymph is pumped through a blood vessel that empties into the body cavity. Hemolymph returns to the blood vessel through openings called ostia. Arthropods like this bee and most mollusks have open circulatory systems.

CIRCULATORY SYSTEM VARIATION IN ANIMALS

The circulatory system varies from simple systems in invertebrates to more complex systems in vertebrates. The simplest animals, such as the sponges (Porifera) and rotifers (Rotifera), do not need a circulatory system because diffusion allows adequate exchange of water, nutrients, and waste, as well as dissolved gases. Organisms that are more complex but still only have two layers of cells in their body plan, such as jellies (Cnidaria) and comb jellies (Ctenophora) also use diffusion through their epidermis and internally through the gastrovascular compartment. Both their internal and external tissues are bathed in an aqueous environment and exchange fluids by diffusion on both sides. Exchange of fluids is assisted by the pulsing of the jellyfish body.

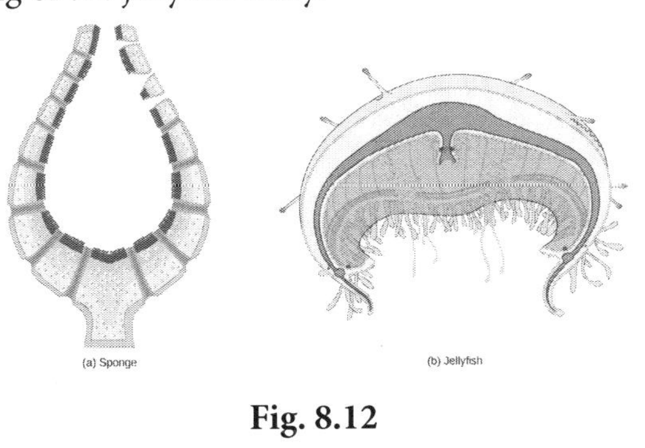

Fig. 8.12

Simple animals consisting of a single cell layer such as the (a) sponge or only a few cell layers such as the (b) jellyfish do not have a circulatory system. Instead, gases, nutrients, and wastes are exchanged by diffusion.

For more complex organisms, diffusion is not efficient for cycling gases, nutrients, and waste effectively through the body; therefore, more complex circulatory systems evolved. In an open system, an elongated beating heart pushes the hemolymph through the body and muscle contractions help to move fluids. The larger more complex crustaceans, including lobsters, have developed arterial-like vessels to push blood through their bodies, and the most active mollusks, such as squids, have evolved a closed circulatory system and are able to move rapidly to catch prey. Closed circulatory systems are a characteristic of vertebrates; however, there are significant differences in the structure of the heart and the circulation of blood between the different vertebrate groups due to adaptation during evolution and associated differences in anatomy. The figure below illustrates the basic circulatory systems of some vertebrates: fish, amphibians, reptiles, and mammals.

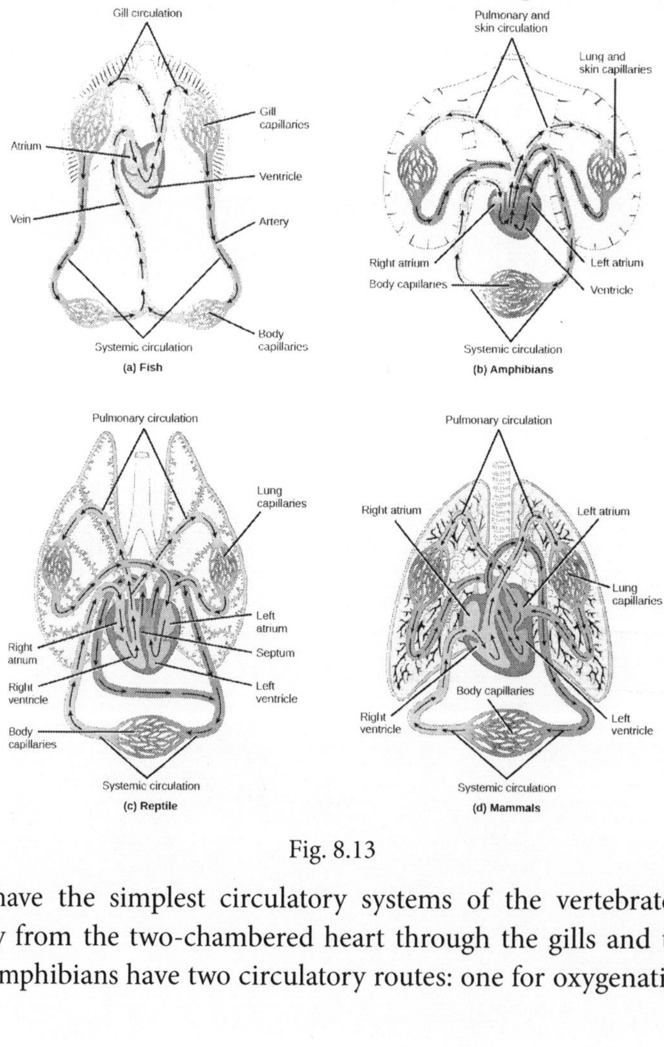

Fig. 8.13

(a) Fish have the simplest circulatory systems of the vertebrates: blood flows unidirectionally from the two-chambered heart through the gills and then the rest of the body. (b) Amphibians have two circulatory routes: one for oxygenation of the blood through the lungs and skin, and the other to take oxygen to the rest of the body. The blood is pumped from a three-chambered heart with two atria and a single ventricle. (c) Reptiles also have two circulatory routes; however, blood is only oxygenated through the lungs. The heart is three chambered, but the ventricles are partially separated so some mixing of oxygenated and deoxygenated blood occurs except in crocodilians and birds. (d) Mammals and birds have the most efficient heart with four chambers that completely separate the oxygenated and deoxygenated blood; it pumps only oxygenated blood through the body and deoxygenated blood to the lungs.

Fish have a single circuit for blood flow and a two-chambered heart that has only a single atrium and a single ventricle. The atrium collects blood that has returned from the body and the ventricle pumps the blood to the gills where gas exchange occurs and the blood is re-oxygenated; this is called gill circulation. The blood then continues through the rest of the body before arriving back at the atrium; this is called systemic circulation. This unidirectional flow of blood produces a gradient of oxygenated to deoxygenated blood around the fishâ€™s systemic circuit. The result is a limit in the amount of oxygen that can reach some of the organs and tissues of the body, reducing the overall metabolic capacity of fish.

In amphibians, reptiles, birds, and mammals, blood flow is directed in two circuits: one through the lungs and back to the heart, which is called pulmonary circulation, and the other throughout the rest of the body and its organs including the brain (systemic circulation). In amphibians, gas exchange also occurs through the skin during pulmonary circulation and is referred to as pulmocutaneous circulation.

Amphibians have a three-chambered heart that has two atria and one ventricle rather than the two-chambered heart of fish. The two atria (superior heart chambers) receive blood from the two different circuits (the lungs and the systems), and then there is some mixing of the blood in the heart's ventricle (inferior heart chamber), which reduces the efficiency of oxygenation. The advantage to this arrangement is that high pressure in the vessels pushes blood to the lungs and body. The mixing is mitigated by a ridge within the ventricle that diverts oxygen-rich blood through the systemic circulatory system and deoxygenated blood to the pulmocutaneous circuit. For this reason, amphibians are often described as having double circulation.

Most reptiles also have a three-chambered heart similar to the amphibian heart that directs blood to the pulmonary and systemic circuits. However, the ventricle is divided more effectively by a partial septum, which results in less mixing of oxygenated and deoxygenated blood. Some reptiles (alligators and crocodiles) are the most "primitive" animals to exhibit a four-chambered heart. Crocodilians have a unique circulatory mechanism where the heart shunts blood from the lungs toward the stomach and other organs during long periods of submergence, for instance, while the animal waits for prey or stays underwater waiting for prey to rot. One adaptation includes two main arteries that leave the same part of the heart: one takes blood to the lungs and the other provides an alternate route to the stomach and other parts of the body. Two other adaptations include a hole in the heart between the two ventricles, called the foramen of Panizza, which allows blood to move from one side of the heart to the other, and specialized connective tissue that slows the blood flow to the lungs.

In mammals and birds, the heart is divided completely into four chambers: two atria and two ventricles. Oxygenated blood is fully separated from deoxygenated blood, which improves the efficiency of double circulation and is probably required for supporting the warm-blooded lifestyle of mammals and birds. The four-chambered heart of birds and mammals evolved independently from a three-chambered heart. The independent evolution of the same or a similar biological trait is referred to as convergent evolution.

Healthy bovine heart

Slightly >10% of all domestic animals examined by a veterinarian have some form of cardiovascular disease (clinically significant or insignificant), with varying prevalences of cardiac disease based on species, breed, and etiology (congenital vs acquired cardiovascular disease). The true prevalence of cardiovascular disease is likely underestimated because the majority of domestic animals do not receive a cardiac workup.

Similar to many chronic diseases of other organ systems, cardiovascular diseases generally do not resolve but progress and become more limiting over time, which may ultimately lead to death. Evaluation of the heart is performed via assessment of:

- heart sounds and murmurs
- arterial pulses
- degree of jugular vein distention
- strength and location of the apex beat
- electrocardiography
- radiography
- cardiac biomarkers
- echocardiography
- other advanced imaging techniques, such as
- angiography
- fluoroscopy
- CT scan with angiography
- cardiac MRI
- Heart Rate and the Electrocardiogram
- ECG, dog

The sinoatrial (SA) node is the pacemaker of the heart. The heartbeat originates with a wave of depolarization that begins in the SA node at the juncture of the cranial vena cava and the right atrium. At rest, the SA node discharges ~30 times/min in horses, >120 times/min in cats (typically 180–220 times/min in a hospital setting), and 60–120 times/min in dogs (range of 40–260 bpm, with average daily rate of 80 bpm for an adult dog based on 24-hour Holter monitoring), depending on their size. In general, the larger the species, the slower the rate of SA node discharge and the slower the heart rate. Birds can have a resting heart rate of ~115–130 beats/min, with active heart rates up to 670 beats/min, depending on size and species. Hummingbirds can have an active heart rate of >1,200 beats/min.

The rate of SA nodal discharge increases when norepinephrine (released from the sympathetic nerves) or epinephrine (released from the adrenal medulla) binds to the beta1-adrenoreceptors on the SA node (sympathetic stimulation). This cardioacceleration (positive chronotropic effect) may be blocked by beta-adrenergic blocking agents (eg, propranolol, atenolol, metoprolol, esmolol, carvedilol). The rate of SA nodal discharge decreases when acetylcholine released by the parasympathetic (vagus) nerves binds to the cholinergic receptors on the SA node (vagal stimulation). This vagally mediated cardiodeceleration (negative chronotropic effect) may be blocked by a parasympatholytic (vagolytic) compound (eg, atropine, glycopyrrolate). When the SA node discharges and the wave of depolarization traverses the atria via preferential pathways (interatrial, internodal, and atrionodal) toward the atrioventricular (AV) node, the P wave (atriogram) of the ECG is produced. Subsequently, the atria contract, ejecting a small volume of remaining blood into the respective ventricles (atrial kick). Atrial repolarization (Ta) is typically difficult to visualize in small animals due to its low voltage deflection.

In quiet, healthy animals, the cyclic variation of the heart rate with respiration is termed respiratory sinus arrhythmia (RSA); it results from decreased vagal activity during inspiration (increase in SA node discharge rate with resultant increase in heart rate) and increased vagal activity during expiration (decrease in SA node discharge rate with resultant decrease in heart rate). In addition to variations in vagal tone with respiration, other mechanisms contribute to RSA, including response of the cardiopulmonary and baroreceptors (eg, Frank-Starling mechanism, Bainbridge reflex). Therefore, vagolytic compounds, as well as excitement, pain, fever, and congestive heart failure (CHF), usually abolish or diminish RSA. Heart rate variability synchronized with respirations is a good indicator of cardiac health. It is rare to find an animal that has active CHF with RSA; however, comorbid conditions that increase vagal activity (such as primary respiratory or neurologic disease) may cause RSA to persist. RSA is uncommonly documented in cats in the hospital setting due to their higher sympathetic tone.

Heart rate is also inversely related to systemic arterial blood pressure. When blood pressure increases, heart rate decreases; when blood pressure decreases, heart rate increases. This relation is known as Marey's Law and occurs by the following mechanism.

When high-pressure arterial baroreceptors in the aortic and carotid sinuses detect increases in blood pressure, they send increased afferent volleys to the medulla oblongata, which increases vagal efferents to the SA node and causes the heart rate to decrease. In heart failure, the baroreceptors (laden with Na+/K+-ATPase) become fatigued, which reduces the afferent signals to the medulla oblongata. This results in less vagal efferent signaling. Thus, dogs in CHF have a decrease in heart rate variability and frequently present with an underlying sinus tachycardia.

Once the wave of depolarization reaches the atrioventricular (AV) node, the speed of conduction is slowed through the nodal tissue, giving the atria time to contract and eject more blood into the ventricles, allowing for atrioventricular synchrony. The depolarization then travels rapidly via a specialized conduction system (ie, bundle of His, right and left bundles branches, Purkinje network) to the subendocardium of the ventricles and to the ventricular septum. From these points, it travels slowly through the ventricular myocardium (subendocardial to epicardial in category A species), producing the QRS complex of the ECG (representing ventricular depolarization) with subsequent mechanical ventricular contraction.

The process of ventricular activation varies between domestic mammals, which are characterized as either category A (dog, human, monkey, cat, rat) or category B (goat, horse, cow, pig, sheep) based on the time and order of the 3 fronts (waves) of depolarization. Animals in category B have more extensive Purkinje fiber networks throughout the ventricular myocardium into the epicardium, thus the wave front does not spread from endocardium to epicardium as in category A mammals. For this reason, chamber enlargement cannot be determined from a base apex lead used for horses and large animals, and the ECG is only used to assess the cardiac rhythm. The delay between the electrical activity visualized on ECG and mechanical function accounts for transmission of impulses, which allows contraction of cardiomyocytes to occur in synchrony. Under rare conditions, there may be depolarization without contraction; this is called electromechanical dissociation.

The interval on an ECG between the onset of the P wave and the onset of the QRS complex is termed the PQ or PR interval. It is a measure of the time it takes for the electrical wave of depolarization to begin at the SA node, traverse the AV node, and reach the ventricles. Factors that speed or slow the rate of discharge of the SA node (chronotropy) also speed or slow conduction through the AV node (dromotropy). Thus, as the heart rate increases, the PR interval shortens; when heart rate slows, the PR interval lengthens.

The T wave of the ECG represents repolarization of the ventricles. It is affected by electrolyte imbalance (eg, hypo- or hyperkalemia, hypo- or hypercalcemia), myocardial injury, or ventricular enlargement. Repolarization of the atria (Ta wave) is rarely seen, because it occurs during the much larger QRS complex. Occasionally, it can be seen with AV nodal disease (AV block) or in horses with slow heart rates, appearing as a "hammock" after the P wave.

The electrocardiogram can be studied in three different anatomic planes, including frontal plane or X-axis of the Cartesian system, sagittal plane or Y-axis of the Cartesian system, and horizontal (transverse) plane or Z-axis of the Cartesian system. In addition, there are three main lead systems used in veterinary medicine for category A mammals: Bailey's hexaxial system (records electrical activity in frontal plane), precordial or chest lead system (records electrical activity in horizontal plane), and bipolar orthogonal system (records electrical activity in all three planes). In category B mammals, a base-apex lead configuration is used. Interpretation of ECGs should be performed in a systematic manner, including assessment of the heart rate and rhythm, evaluating waveforms (P, QRS, T) and segments (PR/PR, ST, QT), and assessing for presence of a P wave for every QRS wave and vice versa. An in-depth review of ECG interpretation is beyond the scope of this discussion.

Force of Ventricular Contraction

The force with which the ventricles contract is determined by many factors, including the end-diastolic volume (preload), which is the volume of blood within the ventricles just before they begin to contract, and myocardial contractility (inotropy), which is the rate of cycling of the microscopic contractile units of the myocardium.

The preload is determined by the difference in end-diastolic pressure between the ventricle and the pleural space, divided by the stiffness of the ventricular myocardium. The end-diastolic pressure of the ventricle is determined by the ratio of blood volume and the compliance of the myocardium. Preload is regulated predominantly by low-pressure volume receptors in the heart and large veins. When these receptors are stimulated by an increase in blood volume or by distention of the structures the receptors occupy, the body responds by making more urine and by dilating the veins—an attempt to decrease blood volume and lower the pressures in the veins responsible for venous distention. An increase in end-diastolic volume (preload) stretches the ventricular wall, resulting in a more forceful contraction as per the Frank-Starling mechanism, or Starling's law of the heart.

Stretching of receptors in the atria and ventricles causes them to release natriuretic proteins: brain natriuretic peptide (BNP) primarily from the ventricles and atrial natriuretic peptide (ANP) from the atria. These peptides are natriuretic, relax smooth muscle, and in general oppose vasopressin and angiotensin II. A correlation between BNP and NT-proBNP levels and degree of stretch of the heart has been identified in dogs.

Myocardial contractility is determined by the availability of ATP and calcium, which allows myosin-actin cross-bridging to occur. The rate of liberation of energy from ATP is determined, in part, by the amount of norepinephrine binding to beta1-adrenergic receptors in the myocardium. One of the most important factors in heart failure is the down-regulation (decreased number) of myocardial beta1-receptors.

Oxygen and the Myocardium

Oxygen is essential for the production of energy that permits all body functions. The amount of oxygen available for production of this energy is termed the tissue oxygen content. The myocardial oxygen content is a balance between how much oxygen is delivered to the heart minus how much oxygen is consumed by the heart.

The amount of oxygen delivered to the heart depends on how well the lungs function, how much Hgb is present to carry the oxygen, and how much blood carrying the Hgb flows through the heart muscle via the coronary arteries. If pulmonary function is normal and there is sufficient Hgb, coronary blood flow will determine how much oxygen is delivered to the myocardium. Coronary blood flow is determined by the difference in mean pressure between the aorta (normally 100 mm Hg) and the right atrium (normally 5 mm Hg), into which coronary blood empties. Because coronary flow is greatest during diastole, slower heart rates (which preferentially increase diastolic interval) are associated with improved myocardial oxygen delivery.

The amount of oxygen consumed by the heart is termed myocardial oxygen consumption. It is determined, principally, by wall tension and heart rate. Wall tension is expressed by the law of LaPlace, in which tension increases with increases in pressure or diameter of the ventricle, and tension decreases with increases in wall thickness of the ventricle. Tension increases with conditions that increase afterload (pressure), such as pulmonary valve stenosis, subaortic stenosis, systemic or pulmonary hypertension, or preload (volume), including mitral valve insufficiency, left-to-right shunting defects, and dilated cardiomyopathy. In the absence of a stenotic lesion, afterload is determined by the relative stiffness of the arteries and by the degree of constriction of the arterioles. The tone of vascular smooth muscle depends on many factors, some of which constrict the muscle (eg, adrenergic agonists, angiotensin II, vasopressin, endothelin) and some of which relax the muscle (eg, norepinephrine, atriopeptin, bradykinin, adenosine, nitric oxide). Afterload is often increased in heart failure, and therapy is often directed at decreasing it.

Increases in heart rate result in increasing myocardial oxygen consumption while decreasing time for diastole when coronary blood flow is greatest. The combination can set the stage for an imbalance in myocardial oxygen demand and supply, leading to myocardial ischemia. Cardiac failure is characterized by an increase in sympathetic tone and relative increases in heart rate; the ultimate impact is an inefficient myocardium that can result in deleterious remodeling.

Oxygen is responsible for the production of the vast majority of ATP, which fuels both contraction and relaxation of the myocardium. Calcium must rapidly be released by intracellular stores (sarcoplasmic reticulum) via calcium-induced calcium release to allow for excitation-contraction coupling, while equally rapid removal of calcium back into the sarcoplasmic reticulum is necessary for relaxation. Both processes of calcium cycling are energy dependent.

In heart failure and cardiomyopathy, inappropriate handling of calcium may result in arrhythmogenesis and may also be the most important factor that leads to both reduced force of contraction and reduced rate of relaxation (ie, reduced systolic as well as diastolic function).

Hindrance to Blood Flow

Blood flow from the heart, termed cardiac output, is via both the left and right ventricles. Cardiac output is determined by the heart rate and ventricular stroke volume. Blood flows through the systemic arterial (left ventricular) or pulmonary arterial (right ventricular) trees and is critical to satisfactory function of the heart and consequent perfusion of organs with adequate quantities of blood and the oxygen it contains. Normal cardiac output for dogs and cats is 100–200 mL/kg/min and 120 mL/kg/min, respectively.

Most (>90%) of the hindrance to blood flow is from the degree of constriction of the arterioles, termed vascular resistance; however, some interference is from the stiffness of the portion of the great arteries closest to the ventricles, termed impedance. Impedance is the sum of external factors opposing left ventricular ejection and is closely related to afterload. The ventricles eject a stroke volume into the proximal portion of the great arteries, which expand to accommodate the stroke volume; when the ventricles are relaxed, the distended great arteries recoil and keep blood moving through the arterioles into the capillaries. The aortic and pulmonic valves close and prevent the stroke volume from returning to the ventricle that ejected it.

Systemic vascular resistance is the opposing blood flow that must be overcome to push blood through the peripheral circulation and is calculated by: (mean arterial pressure – central venous pressure)/cardiac output

Right atrial pressure can also used in place of central venous pressure to calculate systemic vascular resistance. Pulmonary vascular resistance is similarly calculated: (mean pulmonary artery pressure - pulmonary arterial wedge pressure)/cardiac output. Left atrial pressure can be substituted for pulmonary arterial wedge pressure. Pulmonary vascular resistance is increased in cases of pulmonary vascular obstruction or pulmonary hypertension.

One of the most important features of heart failure that leads to morbidity is increased resistance of arterial, arteriolar, and venous smooth muscle because of increased angiotensin II, vasopressin, and endothelin. If the left ventricle is unable to eject a normal stroke volume or cardiac output, it is reasonable that ventricular function might be improved by decreasing vascular resistance. Decreasing afterload (arterial vasodilation) is one therapeutic goal in heart failure therapy.

Valvular heart disease (VHD)

Valvular heart disease (VHD) encompasses a range of cardiovascular conditions, accounting for 10–20% of all cardiac surgeries in the United States 18. As the ageing population continues to increase, so does the prevalence of patients with degenerative valve disorders. In addition, the morbidity and mortality rates of open-heart surgery, the main approach taken for patients with VHD, can be high, providing challenges to reconstructive procedures. Better understanding of the function of the valves and the perturbations that lead to disease is imperative to the future provision of surgical and therapeutic interventions.

There are four cardiac valves: the mitral (bicuspid) valve and aortic semilunar valve on the left side of the heart, and the tricuspid valve and pulmonary semilunar valve on the right side. The heart valve leaflet structure consists of cellular and extracellular components. Extracellular components include collagen, glycosaminoglycans (GAGs) and elastin present in the three layers of the valve: the fibrosa, spongiosa and ventricularis, respectively. Valve surface endothelial cells (VECs) and the inner valve interstitial cells (VICs) are the principal cell types found in the cardiac valves 19, 20, 23.

Simplified cross section of the aortic valve showing progression of aortic valve calcification. Valve endothelial cells (VECs) line the valve leaflet surface. The inner layers of the valve consist of the fibrosa, spongiosa and ventricularis. The principal cell type within each layer is the valve interstitial cells (VICs). The fibrosa contains collagen (Types I and III), the spongiosa contains glycosaminoglycans (GAGs) and the ventricularis—elastin fibres. In calcific aortic valve disease (CAVD), often the fibrosa layer becomes calcified and thickened. This may be because of lipid deposition and inflammatory processes which trigger the osteochondrogenic transdifferentiation of VICs. Calcium deposition then occurs, forming bone-like material as neovascularization around the calcified lesions and remodelling of the extracellular matrix occurs. This results in the formation of calcified nodules and the thickening of the valve leaflet

Over 60% of valve disease mortality is because of semilunar valve dysfunction, especially of the aortic valve, with approximately 50 000 valve replacement or repair procedures reported each year in the USA. Semilunar valve diseases affect all ages, from congenital valve defects in neonates and children, to the increasing number of elderly with calcified valves. These dysfunctional heart valves most often require surgical replacement using mechanical or bioprosthetic valves which are prone to failure over time from structural or thrombosis-related problems.

Although many studies into valvular biology use adult aortic valve tissues and cells from either humans or animals, it is clear that the subject's age is important in order to assess age-specific pathologies and conditions. An earlier study reported numerous age-related changes in the extracellular matrix (ECM) composition and mechanical properties of the aortic valves, in addition to valve cell phenotypes. The ECM is the cell-synthesized structural backbone of connective tissue. It provides a structural frame for mesenchyme-derived tissues, in addition to regulating interactions between numerous growth factors and cell surface receptors. Within the ECM are elastic fibres, collagen fibrils and microfibrils, which contain components including elastin, collagen and the fibrillins. In the cardiovascular system, this complex meshwork also ensures normal cardiovascular function by providing the biomechanical characteristics of the blood vessel walls. Substantial tissue growth and remodelling occur before adulthood. In foetal development, trilaminate ECM structures or highly aligned elastin and collagen that are evident in adult valves are not yet present in the aortic valves. The ECM is also an essential component in the cardiac valves, where its disruption has been reported in valve diseases, as will be mentioned later on. As valvular diseases continue to increase in the elderly population, improving our understanding of how valve cells and the ECM functions change throughout ageing is crucial, as well as distinguishing their responses to surrounding environments in various physiological states, such as those pertaining to vascular calcification.

The function of the cardiac valves is of crucial importance. However, the aortic valve is especially vital as it is a partition between the left ventricle and the aorta, at the level where the coronary arteries arise. Therefore, significant clinical complications occur when congenital defects and chronic disorders relating to the aortic valve are present, as current diagnostic and therapeutic strategies are inadequate. Although there have been major advancements in the last decade or so in valvular biology, there are still many pieces to be found to form a clear picture of the pathological mechanisms that impair valvular function.

MODELS OF CALCIFIC AORTIC VALVE DISEASE

Calcific aortic valve disease (CAVD) is a progressive disorder involving valve leaflet thickening (aortic sclerosis), leading to severe calcification with impaired leaflet motion (aortic stenosis). Aortic stenosis is a major form of CVD, along with hypertension and coronary artery disease, in the Western world. Almost 30% of adults above 65 years have aortic stenosis, and approximately 50% in those above 85 years. It develops from progressive leaflet calcification, causing gradual restriction of the opening of the leaflets. Aortic stenosis shares similarities with atherosclerosis, for example, their risk factors include age, diabetes, hypertension, obesity, increased low-density lipoprotein (LDL) cholesterol and lipoprotein(a), as well as smoking. Pathological studies of human aortic stenosis have identified valvular lesions containing inflammatory cells and calcific deposits similar to those found in atherosclerotic plaques. Once symptoms develop as a result of increasing stenosis severity, including angina and heart failure, there is a higher risk of sudden death with the average survival of only 2–3 years.

Studies assessing the biological and structural changes in aortic valves have predominantly used mouse models. Techniques used have included staining for calcium deposition, quantitative real-time PCR (qRT-PCR) to examine changes in mRNA levels for specific genes, protein quantification and enzymatic activity 36. To date, there are reports of pro-osteogenic signalling cascades thought to contribute to the initiation and progression of aortic stenosis. Signalling molecules include bone morphogenetic proteins (BMPs), Wnt/β-catenin and transforming growth factor-β (TGF-β) although the role of TGF-β in osteogenic signalling is not clear. The RANK/RANKL/OPG pathway is also thought to be involved in the calcification process, which involves complex interactions between receptor activator of nuclear factor kappa B (RANK), RANK ligand (RANKL), and osteoprotegerin (OPG). Matrix remodelling may also be involved in the expansion of calcified plaques and pro-inflammatory processes, through alterations in matrix metalloproteinases (MMPs) and elastin fragments produced by cathepsins 36. Furthermore, the NOTCH1 pathway has been implicated as a regulator of valve calcification, through the repression of the osteoblast transcription factor Runt-related transcription factor 2 (RUNX2). This suggests an inhibitory role of NOTCH1 in valvular calcification. Additionally, a number of ECM proteins have been found to have roles in CAVD including collagen, elastin and GAGs, where changes in their expression have impacts on cellular processes, and also cause valve leaflet thickening 39.

Simplified diagram showing potential RANK/RANKL/OPG involvement in bone remodelling and in vascular calcification. Receptor activator of nuclear factor kappa-B ligand (RANKL) from osteoblasts or endothelial cells binds to the Receptor Activator of Nuclear Factor kappa-B (RANK) of osteoclast precursors, or vascular smooth muscle cells (VSMCs). This leads to differentiation into mature osteoclasts in the bone, which are involved in bone resorption, whereas in vascular calcification, VSMCs undergo a phenotypic transition into osteochondrogenic cells that can deposit mineralized matrix. Osteoprotegerin (OPG) is the decoy receptor for RANKL, and a potential inhibitor for mineralization

Simplified diagram showing potential NOTCH1 involvement in vascular calcification. NOTCH1 signalling may be involved in the inhibition, as well as the promotion, of vascular calcification through additional factors. Black arrows indicate stimulatory effects, whilst red lines indicate inhibitory effects.

Pro-mineralization processes can also be regulated by circulating calcification inhibitors, including matrix γ-carboxyglutamic acid or matrix Gla protein (MGP), which inhibits BMP signalling 40. CAVD patients were also found to have less circulating MGP 41. Another circulating inhibitor of calcification, Fetuin-A, binds clusters of calcium and phosphate, preventing their uptake into cells. Circulating levels of Fetuin-A have been shown to be reduced in peritoneal dialysis patients displaying rapid development of valvular calcification. Furthermore a cross-sectional study of 970 patients with coronary artery disease found an inverse relationship between circulating Fetuin-A levels and mitral and aortic valve calcification. Aortic stenosis in patients with CAVD has also been associated with increased plasma levels of potential promoters of calcification, such as the non-collagenous bone matrix protein osteopontin (OPN), a pro-inflammatory glycoprotein that regulates calcium deposition by osteoblasts.

The mechanism for CAVD development is similar to skeletal bone formation (ossification). CAVD progression is regulated by cells within the valve that develop an osteoblast-like phenotype 46. Within calcified aortic valves, markers of bone differentiation have also been discovered, including RUNX2, OPN, osteocalcin (OCN) and bone sialoprotein. RUNX2 expression is a marker for osteoblast differentiation, whilst OCN is a late marker of calcification in osteoblastogenesis. Intriguingly, ossification, the active process of bone tissue repair and remodelling, is observed in end-stage VHD 50. In addition to the presence of mature lamellar bone and infiltration of inflammatory cells, BMPs -2 and -4 have been found in calcified valves 50. BMP-2 is a potent osteogenic differentiation marker, a member of the TGF-β superfamily, and has been found to be involved in calcification following the repression of NOTCH1 signalling in sheep aortic VICs. Mutations in NOTCH1 have been linked with the presence of aortic valve calcification in human and mouse studies, although the disease was much milder in the latter 51. A recent study of NOTCH1 in human aortic VECs found that this factor positively regulated MGP. Shear stress was simulated by media flow conditions in vitro and was found to activate NOTCH1 expression. Because MGP can inhibit BMPs, this may be the route through which NOTCH1 represses BMP-2. Intriguingly, it has been reported that NOTCH1 induces the differentiation and calcification of vascular smooth muscle cells (VSMCs) through a BMP-2 driven mechanism (Figure (Figure3)3). However, the role of NOTCH1 in the calcification of valves and vessels remains to be fully understood, and requires further investigation.

The mechanisms underpinning the process of valvular calcification have yet to be fully elucidated. However, an 'initiation' and 'propagation' phase has been described. It may be that in response to valvular damage, such as through endothelial disruption via shear stress, lipid deposition and inflammation occur, which subsequently triggers calcification. Neovascularization was also found in calcified valves, suggesting that this is important in CAVD, with new vessels commonly found in areas of inflammation around calcified deposits. Haemorrhage has been associated with neoangiogenesis, macrophage infiltration and accelerated disease progression in patients with advanced aortic stenosis. Nevertheless, the roles of the factors and pathways involved in VHDs and other CVDs, including those briefly mentioned above, remain unclear. More information into the early stages of disease initiation and progression is required to understand the mechanisms of CAVD.

Currently, the only option to treat CAVD is through valve replacement surgery. This reflects our lack of understanding of the early pathobiological processes, even though later stages of the disease are well described. Additionally, as the implicated regulators of ectopic calcification are required for normal bone mineralization, establishing a therapeutic strategy that does not affect bone is crucial. And so, uncovering the factors and mechanisms that are important during the initiation and progression of these diseases facilitated by animal models is required for developing such treatments and interventions. Many studies into aortic stenosis utilize the mouse as a model. However, the size of the aortic valves limits the amount of material available for examining the molecular mechanisms behind CAVD. Although diseased human valve samples can be obtained relatively easily, acquiring healthy samples is nearly impossible. In contrast, healthy valve samples from animals are far more accessible, can be used as a healthy control and can provide a source of valve cells that can be isolated for experimentation.

9

RESPIRATORY SYSTEM

The respiratory system (also respiratory apparatus, ventilatory system) is a biological system consisting of specific organs and structures used for gas exchange in animals and plants. The anatomy and physiology that make this happen varies greatly, depending on the size of the organism, the environment in which it lives and its evolutionary history. In land animals the respiratory surface is internalized as linings of the lungs. Gas exchange in the lungs occurs in millions of small air sacs; in mammals and reptiles these are called alveoli, and in birds they are known as atria. These microscopic air sacs have a very rich blood supply, thus bringing the air into close contact with the blood. These air sacs communicate with the external environment via a system of airways, or hollow tubes, of which the largest is the trachea, which branches in the middle of the chest into the two main bronchi. These enter the lungs where they branch into progressively narrower secondary and tertiary bronchi that branch into numerous smaller tubes, the bronchioles. In birds the bronchioles are termed parabronchi. It is the bronchioles, or parabronchi that generally open into the microscopic alveoli in mammals and atria in birds. Air has to be pumped from the environment into the alveoli or atria by the process of breathing which involves the muscles of respiration.

In most fish, and a number of other aquatic animals (both vertebrates and invertebrates) the respiratory system consists of gills, which are either partially or completely external organs, bathed in the watery environment. This water flows over the gills by a variety of active or passive means. Gas exchange takes place in the gills which consist of thin or very flat filaments and lammelae which expose a very large surface area of highly vascularized tissue to the water.

Other animals, such as insects, have respiratory systems with very simple anatomical features, and in amphibians even the skin plays a vital role in gas exchange. Plants also have respiratory systems but the directionality of gas exchange can be opposite to that in animals. The respiratory system in plants includes anatomical features such as stomata, that are found in various parts of the plant.

RESPIRATION IN ANIMALS

The mode of external respiration varies greatly from organism to organism. The basic process of respiration (cellular respiration) is similar in all living organisms. The process of exchange gases varies in different animals.

1. Through Plasma Membrane

In unicellular animals, such as amoeba, exchange of gases takes place through cell surface. They absorb oxygen from the surrounding air or water and give out carbon dioxide through plasma membrane by diffusion.

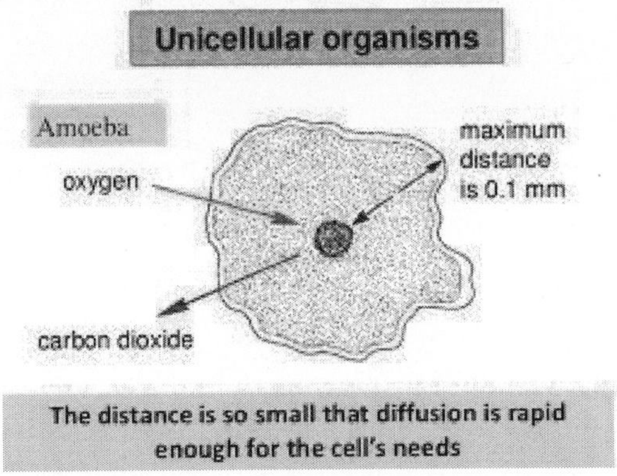

Fig. 9.1

2. Through Body Wall or Skin

Tapeworms, earthworms, and leeches use their skin for the exchange of gases. The skin of Earthworms is very thin and moistened. Many blood cells are spread on this skin. These blood cells are known as capillaries. The exchange of gases occurs at capillaries. They die of suffocation if their skin is dried up.

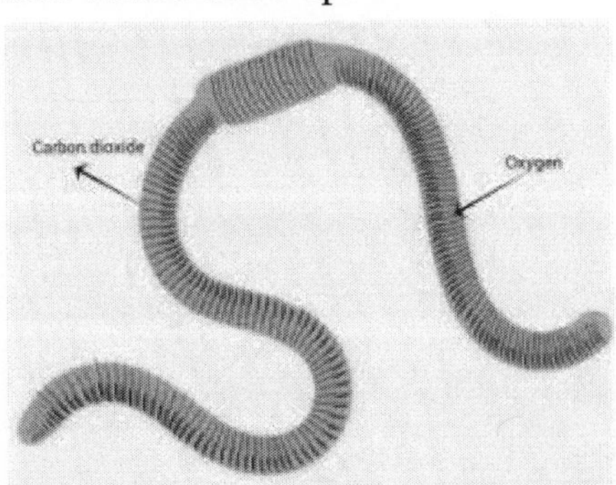

Fig. 9.2

Amphibians such as frogs use more than one organ of respiration during their life. They breathe through gills while they are tadpoles. Mature frogs breathe mainly with lungs and also exchange gas with the environment through skin.

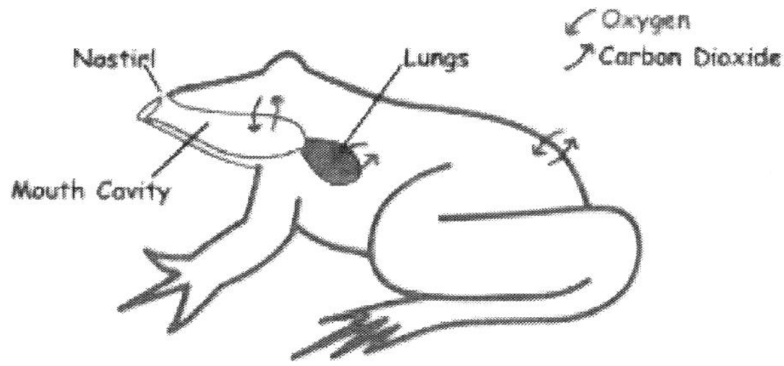

Fig. 9.3

3. Through Tracheal System

In insects like cockroaches, grasshopper, transportation of gas or gaseous exchange take place by a special type of fine tubes is called tracheae.

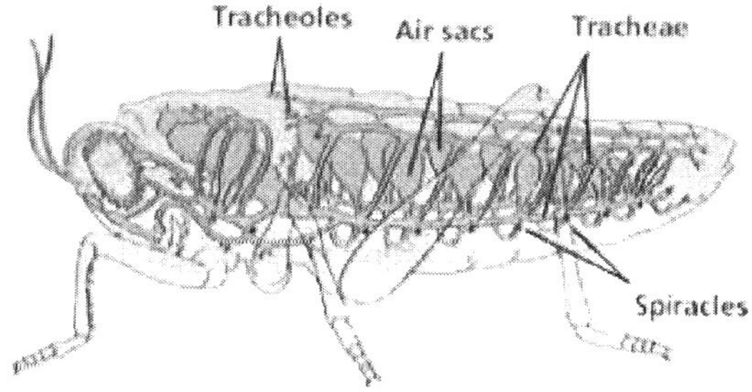

Fig. 9.4

Air containing oxygen enters through spiracles into the tracheal tubes. It then diffuses into the body tissue and reaches every cell in the body. Carbon dioxide released from the cells goes into the tracheal tubes and comes out through spiracles.

4. Through Gills

A majority of aquatic animals like fish and prawns breathe through special organs called gills. Gilla are projections of the skin that help in using oxygen dissolved in water. Gills contain blood vessels which help in exchange of gases.

The gill of fish

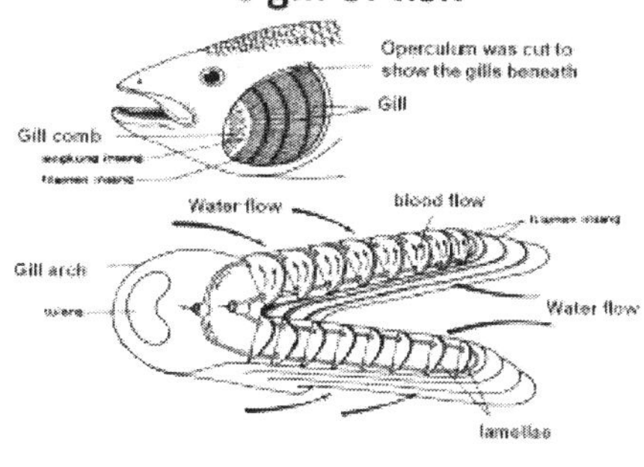

Fig. 9.5

Fish live in water. To get oxygen dissolved in water, fish gulp water through the mouth and pump it over the gills. Water passes into the gill chamber through gill slits. In each chamber, the water passes over the filaments. They absorb oxygen from the water and replace it with carbon dioxide formed. The water then passes out through the gill opening and this process is repeated again and again.

5. Through lungs

Amphibians, mammals, and birds exchange gases through special respiratory organs called lungs. Lungs are air-filled sac-like structures in the chest cavity. They are connected to the outside by a series of tubes and small opening.

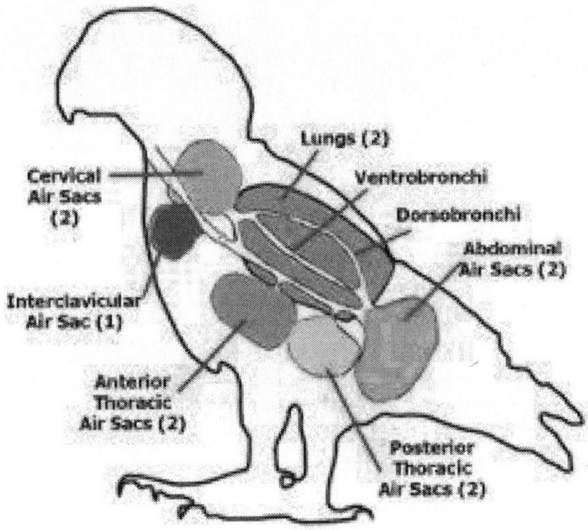

Fig. 9.6

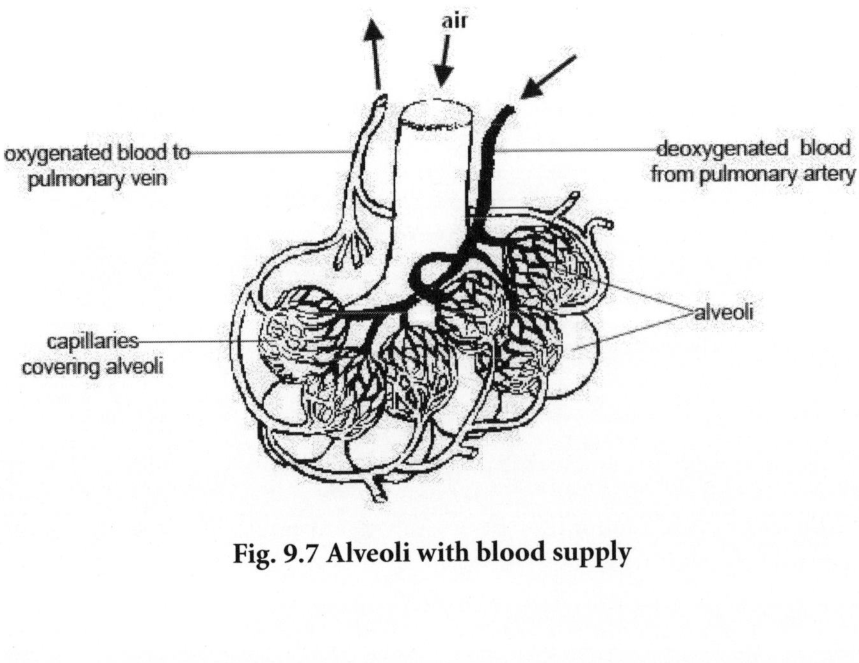

Fig. 9.7 Alveoli with blood supply

Animals require a supply of energy to survive. This energy is needed to build large molecules like proteins and glycogen, make the structures in cells, move chemicals through membranes and around cells, contract muscles, transmit nerve impulses and keep the body warm. Animals get their energy from the large molecules that they eat as food. Glucose is often the energy source but it may also come from other carbohydrates, as well as fats and protein. The energy is made by the biochemical process known as cellular respiration that takes place in the mitochondria inside every living cell.

The overall reaction can be summarised by the word equation given below. Charbohydrate Food (glucose) + Oxygen = Carbon Dioxide + Water + energy As you can see from this equation, the cells need to be supplied with oxygen and glucose and the waste product, carbon dioxide , which is poisonous to cells, needs to be removed. The way the digestive system provides the glucose for cellular respiration will be described ("The Gut and Digestion"), but here we are only concerned with the two gases, oxygen and carbon dioxide, that are involved in cellular respiration. These gases are carried in the blood to and from the tissues where they are required or produced.

Oxygen enters the body from the air (or water in fish)and carbon dioxide is usually elimi- nated from the same part of the body. This process is called gas exchange . In fish gas exchange occurs in the gills, in land dwelling vertebrates lungs are the gas exchange organs and frogs use gills when they are tadpoles and lungs, the mouth and the skin when adults.

Mammals (and birds) are active and have relatively high body temperatures so they require large amounts of oxygen to provide sufficient energy through cellular respiration.

DIFFUSION AND TRANSPORT OF OXYGEN

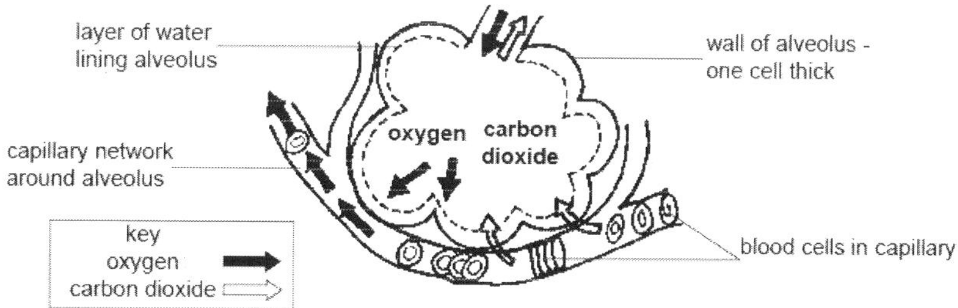

Fig. 9.8

to take in enough oxygen and release all the carbon dioxide produced they need a very large surface area over which gas exchange can take place. The many minute air sacs or alveoli of the lungs provide this. When you look at these under the microscope they appear rather like bunches of grapes covered with a dense network of fine capillaries. A thin layer of water covers the inner surface of each alveolus. There is only a very small distance -just 2 layers of thin cells - between the air in the alveoli and the blood in the capillaries. The gases pass across this gap by diffusion .

1. Diffusion and Transport of Oxygen

The air in the alveoli is rich in oxygen while the blood in the capillaries around the alveoli is deoxygenated. This is because the haemoglobin in the red blood cells has released all the oxygen it has been carrying to the cells of the body. Oxygen diffuses from high concentration to low concentration. It therefore crosses the narrow barrier between the alveoli and the capillaries to enter the blood and combine with the haemoglobin in the red blood cells to form oxyhaemoglobin .

The narrow diameter of the capillaries around the alveoli means that the blood flow is slowed down and that the red cells are squeezed against the capillary walls. Both of these factors help the oxygen diffuse into the blood.

When the blood reaches the capillaries of the tissues the oxygen splits from the haemoglobin molecule. It then diffuses into the tissue fluid and then into the cells.

2. Diffusion and Transport Of Carbon Dioxide

Blood entering the lung capillaries is full of carbon dioxide that it has collected from the tissues. Most of the carbon dioxide is dissolved in the plasma either in the form of sodium bicarbonate or carbonic acid . A little is transported by the red blood cells. As the blood enters the lungs the carbon dioxide gas diffuses through the capillary and alveoli walls into the water film and then into the alveoli. Finally it is removed from the lungs during breathing out.

3. The Air Passages

When air is breathed in it passes from the nose to the alveoli of the lungs down a series of tubes. After entering the nose the air passes through the nasal cavity, which is lined with a moist membrane that adds warmth and moisture to the air as it passes. The air then flows through the pharynx or throat, a passage that carries both food and air, to the larynx where the voice-box is located. Here the passages for food and air separate again. Food must pass into the oesophagus and the air into the windpipe or trachea . To prevent food entering this, a small flap of tissue called the epiglottis closes the opening during swallowing. A reflex that inhibits breathing during swallowing also (usually) prevents choking on food.

The trachea is the tube that ducts the air down the throat. Incomplete rings of cartilage in its walls help keep it open even when the neck is bent and head turned. The fact that acrobats and people that tie themselves in knots doing yoga still keep breathing during the most contorted manoeuvres shows how effective this arrangement is. The air passage now divides into the two bronchi that take the air to the right and left lungs before dividing into smaller and smaller bronchioles that spread throughout the lungs to carry air to the alveoli. Smooth muscles in the walls of the bronchi and bronchioles adjust the diameter of the air passages.

The tissue lining the respiratory passages producesmucus and is covered with minute hairs or cilia. Any dust that is breathed into the respiratory system immediately gets entangled in the mucous and the cilia move it towards the mouth or nose where it can be coughed up or blown out.

4. *The Lungs And The Pleural Cavities*

The lungs fill most of the chest or thoracic cavity , which is completely separated from the abdominal cavity by the diaphragm . The lungs and the spaces in which they lie (called the pleural cavities) are covered with membranes called the pleura . There is a thin film of fluid between the two membranes. This lubricates them as they move over each other during breathing movements.

COLLAPSED LUNGS

The pleural cavities are completely airtight with no connection with the outside and if they are punctured by accident (a broken rib will often do this), air rushes in and the lung collapses. Separating the two lungs is a region of tissue that contains the oesophagus, trachea, aorta, vena cava and lymph nodes. This is called the mediastinum. In humans and sheep it separates the cavity completely so that puncturing one pleural cavity leads to the collapse of only one lung. In dogs, however, this separation is incomplete so a puncture results in a complete collapse of both lungs.

5. *Breathing*

The process of breathing moves air in and out of the lungs. Sometimes this process is called respiration but it is important not to confuse it with the chemical process, cellular respiration , that takes place in the mitochondria of cells. Breathing is brought about by the movement of the diaphragm and the ribs.

INSPIRATION

The diaphragm is a thin sheet of muscle that completely separates the abdominal and thoracic cavities. When at rest it domes up into the thoracic cavity but during breathing in or inspiration it flattens. At the same time special muscles in the chest wall move the ribs forwards and outwards. These movements of both the diaphragm and the ribs cause the volume of the thorax to increase. Because the pleural cavities are airtight, the lungs expand to fill this increased space and air is drawn down the trachea into the lungs.

Expiration

Expiration or breathing out consists of the opposite movements. The ribs move down and in and the diaphragm resumes its domed shape so the air is expelled. Expiration is usually passive and no energy is required (unless you are blowing up a balloon).

Lung Volumes

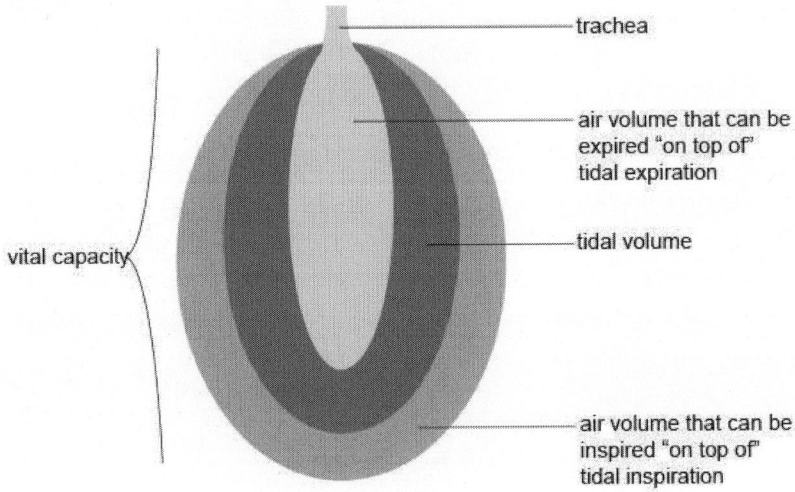

Fig. 9.10 Lung volumes

As you sit here reading this just pay attention to your breathing. Notice that your in and out breaths are really quite small and gentle (unless you have just rushed here from somewhere else!). Only a small amount of the total volume that your lungs hold is breathed in and out with each breath. This kind of gentle "at rest" breathing is called tidal breathing and the volume breathed in or out (they should be the same) is the tidal volume. Sometimes people want to measure the volume of air inspired or expired during a minute of this normal breathing. This is called the minute volume . It could be estimated by measuring the volume of one tidal breath and then multiplying that by the number of breaths in a minute. Of course it is possible to take a deep breath and breathe in as far as you can and then expire as far as possible. The volume of the air expired when a maximum expiration follows a maximum inspiration is called the vital capacity.

COMPOSITION OF AIR

The air animals breathe in consists of 21% oxygen and 0.04% carbon dioxide. Expelled air consists of 16% oxygen and 4.4% carbon dioxide. This means that the lungs remove only a quarter of the oxygen contained in the air. This is why it is possible to give someone (or an animal) artificial respiration by blowing expired air into their mouth.

Breathing is usually an unconscious activity that takes place whether you are awake or asleep, although, humans at least, can also control it consciously. Two regions in the hindbrain called the medulla oblongata and pons control the rate of breathing. These are called respiratory centres . They respond to the concentration of carbon dioxide in the blood. When this concentration rises during a bout of activity, for example, nerve impulses are automatically sent to the diaphragm and rib muscles that increase the rate and the depth of breathing. Increasing the rate of breathing also increases the amount of oxygen in the blood to meet the needs of this increased activity.

The Acidity of the Blood And Breathing

The degree of acidity of the blood (the acid-base balance) is critical for normal functioning of cells and the body as a whole. For example, blood that is too acidic or alkaline can seriously affect nerve function causing a coma, muscle spasms, convulsions and even death. Carbon dioxide carried in the blood makes the blood acidic and the higher the concentration of carbon dioxide the more acidic it is. This is obviously dangerous so there are various mechanisms in the body that bring the acid-base balance back within the normal range. Breathing is one of these homeostatic mechanisms. By increasing the rate of breathing the animal increases the amount of dissolved carbon dioxide that is expelled from the blood. This reduces the acidity of the blood.

BREATHING IN BIRDS

Birds have a unique respiratory system that enables them to respire at the very high rates necessary for flight. The lungs are relatively solid structures that do not change shape and size in the same way as mammalian lungs do. Tubes run through them and connect with a series of air sacs situated in the thoracic and abdominal body cavities and some of the bones. Movements of the ribs and breastbone or sternum expand and compress these air sacs so they act rather like bellows and pump air through the lungs. The evolution of this extremely efficient system of breathing has enabled birds to migrate vast distances and fly at altitudes higher than the summit of Everest.

10

LYMPHATIC SYSTEM

When tissue fluid enters the small blind-ended lymphatic capillaries that form a network between the cells it becomes lymph . Lymph is a clear watery fluid that is very similar to blood plasma except that it contains large numbers of white blood cells, mostly lympho- cytes. It also contains protein, cellular debris, foreign particles and bacteria. Lymph that comes from the intestines also contains many fat globules following the absorption of fat from the digested food into the lymphatics (lacteals) of the villi From the lymph capillaries the lymph flows into larger tubes called lymphatic vessels. These carry the lymph back to join the blood circulation.

LYMPHATIC VESSELS

Lymphatic vessels have several similarities to veins. Both are thin walled and return fluid to the right hand side of the heart. The movement of the fluid in both is brought about by the contraction of the muscles that surround them and both have valves to prevent backflow. One important difference is that lymph passes through at least one lymph node or gland before it reaches the blood system. These filter out used cell parts, cancer cells and bacteria and help defend the body from infection.

Lymph nodes are of various sizes and shapes and found throughout the body. They consist of lymph tissue surrounded by a fibrous sheath. Lymph flows into them through a number of incoming vessels. It then trickles through small channels where white cells called macrophages (derived from monocytes) remove the bacteria and debris by engulfing and digesting them. The lymph then leaves the lymph nodes through outgoing vessels to continue its journey towards the heart where it rejoins the blood circulation.

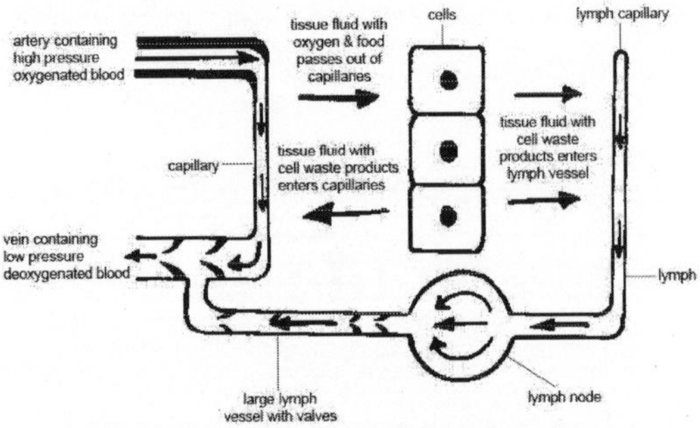

Fig.10.1 The lymphatic system

◉ The circulation of lymph with major lymph nodes

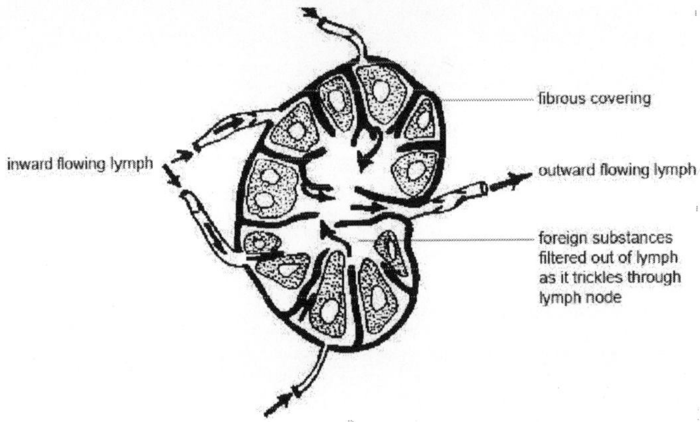

Fig. 10.2 - A lymph node

As well as filtering the lymph, lymph nodes produce the white cells known as lymphocytes. Lymphocytes are also produced by the thymus , spleen and bone marrow . There are two kinds of lymphocyte. The first attach invading micro organisms directly while others produce antibodies that circulate in the blood and attack them.

The function of the lymphatic system can therefore be summarized as transport and defense. It is important for returning the fluid and proteins that have escaped from the blood capillaries to the blood system and is also responsible for picking up the products of fat digestion in the small intestine. Its other essential function is as part of the immune system, defending the body against infection.

Problems with lymph nodes and the lymphatic system

During infection of the body the lymph nodes often become swollen and tender because of their increased activity. This is what causes the swollen 'glands' in your neck during throat infections, mumps and tonsillitis. Sometimes the bacteria multiply in the lymph node and cause inflammation. Cancer cells may also be carried to the lymph nodes and then transported to other parts of the body where they may multiply to form a secondary growth or metastasis. The lymphatic system may therefore contribute to the spread of cancer. Inactivity of the muscles surrounding the lymphatic vessels or blockage of these vessels causes tissue fluid to 'back up' in the tissues resulting in swelling or oedema .

OTHER ORGANS OF THE LYMPHATIC SYSTEM

The spleen is an important part of the lymphatic system. It is a deep red organ situated in the abdomen caudal to the stomach. It is composed of two different types of tissue. The first type makes and stores lymphocytes, the cells of the immune system. The second type of tissue destroys worn out red blood cells, breaking down the haemoglobin into iron, which is recycled, and waste products that are excreted. The spleen also stores red blood cells. When severe blood loss occurs, it contracts and releases them into the circulation.

The thymus is a large pink organ lying just under the sternum (breastbone) just cranial to the heart. It has an important function processing lymphocytes so they are capable of recognising and attacking foreign invaders like bacteria.

Other lymph organs are the bone marrow of the long bones where lymphocytes are pro- duced and lymph nodules , which are like tiny lymph nodes. Large clusters of these are found in the wall of the small intestine (called Peyer's Patches) and in the tonsils.

11

THE GUT AND DIGESTION

Plant cells are made of organic molecules using energy from the sun. This process is called photosynthesis . Animals rely on these ready-made organic molecules to supply them with their food. Some animals (herbivores) eat plants; some (carnivores) eat the herbivores.

HERBIVORES

Herbivoreseat plant material. While no animal produces the digestive enzymes to break down the large cellulose molecules in the plant cell walls, micro-organisms' like bacteria, on the other hand, can break them down. Therefore herbivores employ micro-organisms to do the job for them.

- There are three types of herbivore:
- The first, ruminants like cattle, sheep and goats, house these bacteria in a special com- partment in the enlarged stomach called the rumen .
- The second group has an enlarged large intestine and caecum, called a functional caecum, occupied by cellulose digesting micro-organisms. These non-ruminant herbivores include the horse, rabbit and rat.
- Humans also have a cecum and can be classified as the third type of herbivorous class, along with orangutans and gorillas.

Plants are a primary pure and good source of nutrients, however they are digested very easily and therefore herbivores have to eat large quantities of food to obtain all they require. Herbivores like cows, horses and rabbits typically spend much of their day feeding. To give the micro- organisms access to the cellulose molecules, the plant cell walls need to be broken down. This is why herbivores have teeth that are adapted to crush and grind. Their guts also tend to be lengthy and the food takes a long time to pass through it.

Eating plants have other advantages. Plants are immobile so herbivores normally have to spend little energy collecting them. This contrasts with another main group of animals - the carnivores that often have to chase their prey.

Carnivores

Carnivorous animals like those in the cat and dog families, polar bears, seals, crocodiles and birds of prey catch and eat other animals. They often have to use large amounts of energy finding, stalking, catching and killing their prey. However, they are rewarded by the fact that meat provides a very concentrated source of nutrients. Carnivores in the wild therefore tend to eat distinct meals often with long and irregular intervals between them. Time after feeding is spent digesting and absorbing the food.

The guts of carnivores are usually shorter and less complex than those of herbivores be- cause meat is easier to digest than plant material. Carnivores usually have teeth that are specialised for dealing with flesh, gristle and bone. They have sleek bodies, strong, sharp claws and keen senses of smell, hearing and sight. They are also often cunning, alert and have an aggressive nature.

Omnivores

Many animals feed on both animal and vegetable material – they are omnivorous. Most primates, including humans, are herbivorous but a few, such as chimpanzees belong to this category as do pigs and rats. Their food is diverse, ranging from plant material to animals they have either killed themselves or scavenged from other carnivores. Omnivores lack the specialised teeth and guts of carnivores and herbivores but are often highly intelligent and adaptable reflecting their varied diet.

Treatment Of Food

Whether an animal eats plants or flesh, the carbohydrates , fats and proteins in the food it eats are generally giant molecules. These need to be split up into smaller ones before they can pass into the blood and enter the cells to be used for energy or to make new cell constituents.

For example: Carbohydrates like cellulose, starch, and glycogen need to be split into glucose and other monosaccharides ;

- Proteins need to be split into amino acids ;
- Fats or lipids need to be split into fatty acids and glycerol .

The Gut

The digestive tract, alimentary canal or gut is a hollow tube stretching from the mouth to the anus. It is the organ system concerned with the treatment of foods.

At the mouth the large food molecules are taken into the gut - this is called ingestion. They must then be broken down into smaller ones by digestive enzymes - digestion, before they can be taken from the gut into the blood stream - absorption. The cells of the body can then use these small molecules - assimilation. The indigestible waste products are eliminated from the body by the act of egestion (see diagram 11.1).

1. Transporting the food;
2. Processing the food physically by breaking it up (chewing), mixing, adding fluid etc.
3. Processing the food chemically by adding digestive enzymes to split large food molecules into smaller ones.
4. Absorbing these small molecules into the blood stream so the body can use them.

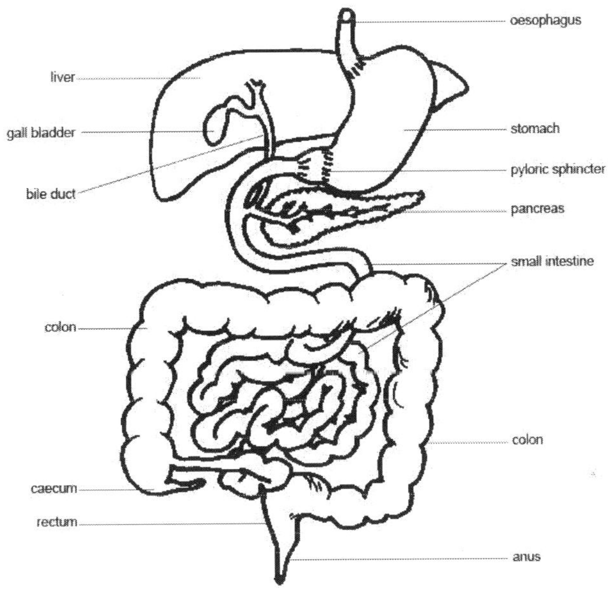

Fig. 11.1 A typical mammalian gut

The food that enters the mouth passes to the oesophagus , then to the stomach , small intestine, cecum , large intestine, rectum and finally undigested material exits at the anus. The liver and pancreas produce secretions that aid digestion and the gall bladder stores bile. Herbivores have an appendix which they use for the digestion of cellulose. Carnivores have an appendix but is not of any function anymore due to the fact that their diet is not based on cellulose anymore.

Mouth

The mouth takes food into the body. The lips hold the food inside the mouth during chewing and allow the baby animal to suck on its mother's teat. In elephants the lips (and nose) have developed into the trunk which is the main food collecting tool. Some mammals, e.g. hamsters, have stretchy cheek pouches that they use to carry food or material to make their nests.

The sight or smell of food and its presence in the mouth stimulates the salivary glands to secrete saliva. There are four pairs of these glands in cats and dogs. The fluid they produce moistens and softens the food making it easier to swallow. It also contains the enzyme, salivary amylase , which starts the digestion of starch.

The tongue moves food around the mouth and rolls it into a ball for swallowing. Taste buds are located on the tongue and in dogs and cats it is covered with spiny projections used for grooming and lapping. The cow's tongue is prehensile and wraps around grass to graze it.

Swallowing is a complex reflex involving 25 different muscles. It pushes food into the oesophagus and at the same time a small flap of tissue called the epiglottis closes off the windpipe so food doesn't go 'down the wrong way' and choke the animal.

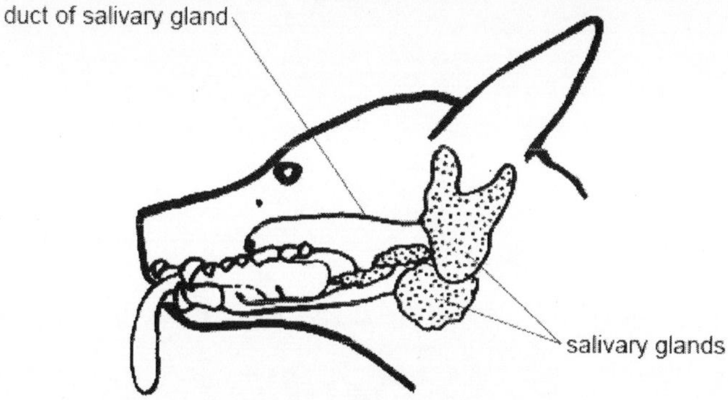

).

Fig. 11.2 a - Salivary glands

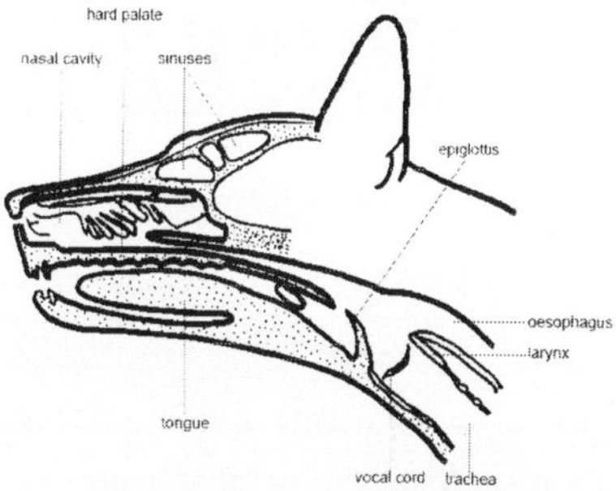

Fig. 11.2 b- Section through the head of a dog

Teeth

Teeth seize, tear and grind food. They are inserted into sockets in the bone and consist of a crown above the gum and root below. The crown is covered with a layer of enamel , the hardest substance in the body. Below this is the dentine , a softer but tough and shock resistant material. At the centre of the tooth is a space filled with pulp which contains blood vessels and nerves. The tooth is cemented into the socket and in most teeth the tip of the root is quite narrow with a small opening for the blood vessels and nerves.

In teeth that grow continuously, like the incisors of rodents, the opening remains large and these teeth are called open rooted teeth. Mammals have 2 distinct sets of teeth. The first the milk teeth are replaced by the permanent teeth .

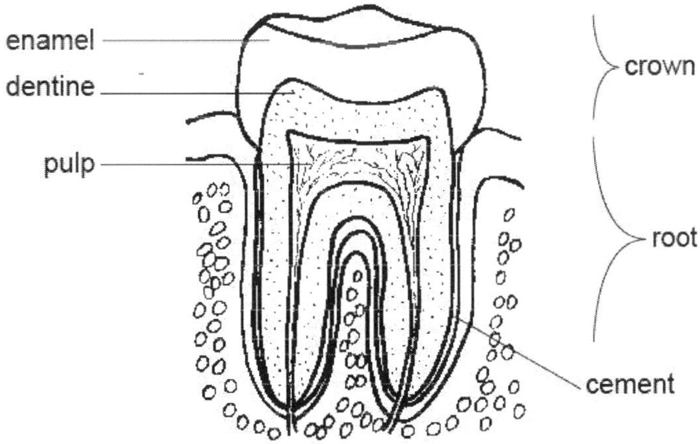

Fig. 11.3 - Structure of a tooth

TYPES OF TEETH

All the teeth of fish and reptiles are similar but mammals usually have four different types of teeth.

The incisors are the chisel-shaped 'biting off' teeth at the front of the mouth. In rodents and rabbits the incisors never stop growing (open-rooted teeth). They must be worn or ground down continuously by gnawing. They have hard enamel on one surface only so they wear unevenly and maintain their sharp cutting edge.

The largest incisors in the animal kingdom are found in elephants, for tusks are actually giant incisors. Sloths have no incisors at all, and sheep have no incisors in the upper jaw. Instead there is a horny pad against which the bottom incisors cut.

The canines or 'wolf-teeth' are long, cone-shaped teeth situated just behind the incisors. They are particularly well developed in the dog and cat families where they are used to hold, stab and kill the prey.

The tusks of boars and walruses are large canines while rodents and herbivores like sheep have no (or reduced) canines. In these animals the space where the canines would normally be is called the diastema. In rodents like the rat and beaver it allows the debris from gnawing to be expelled easily.

The cheek teeth or premolars and molars crush and grind the food. They are particularly well developed in herbivores where they have complex ridges that form broad grinding surfaces. These are created from alternating bands of hard enamel and softer dentine that wear at different rates.

In carnivores the premolars and molars slice against each other like scissors and are called carnassial teeth. They are used for shearing flesh and bone.

DENTAL FORMULA

The numbers of the different kinds of teeth can be expressed in a dental formula. This gives the numbers of incisors, canines, premolars and molars in one half of the mouth. The numbers of these four types of teeth in the left or right half of the upper jaw are written above a horizontal line and the four types of teeth in the right or left half of the lower jaw are written below it.

Thus the dental formula for the sheep is: 0.0.3.3

It indicates that in the upper right (or left) half of the jaw there are no incisors or canines (*i.e.* there is a diastema), three premolars and three molars. In the lower right (or left) half of the jaw are three incisors, one canine, three premolars and three molars.

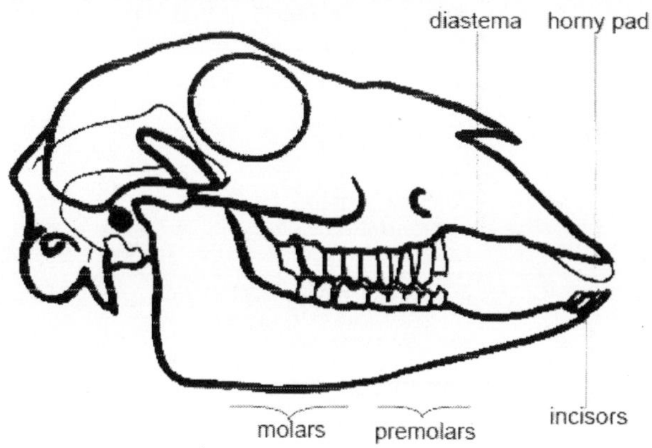

Fig. 11.4

The formula indicates that in the right (or left) half of the upper jaw there are three incisors, one canine, four premolars and two molars. In the right (or left) half of the lower jaw there are three incisors, one canine, four premolars and three molars.

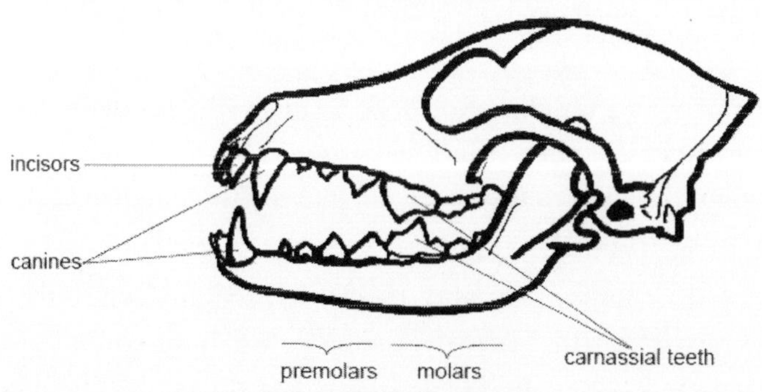

Fig. 11.5 A dog's skull

Oesophagus

The oesophagus transports food to the stomach. Food is moved along the oesophagus, as it is along the small and large intestines, by contraction of the smooth muscles in the walls that push the food along rather like toothpaste along a tube. This movement is called peristalsis.

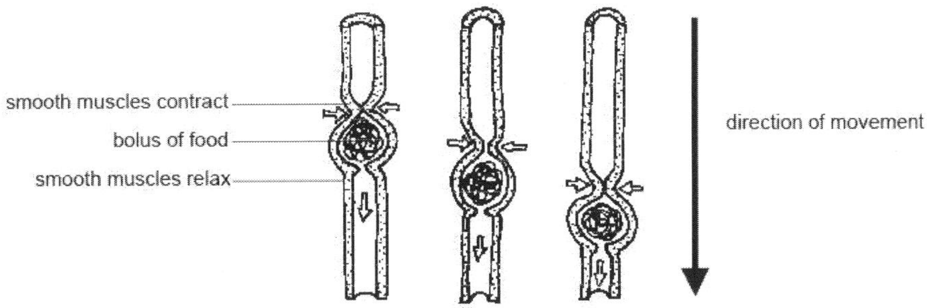

Fig. 11.6 - Peristalsis

Stomach

The stomach stores and mixes the food. Glands in the wall secrete gastric juice that contains enzymes to digest protein and fats as well as hydrochloric acid to make the contents very acidic. The walls of the stomach are very muscular and churn and mix the food with the gastric juice to form a watery mixture called chyme (pronounced kime). Rings of muscle called sphincters at the entrance and exit to the stomach control the movement of food into and out of it.

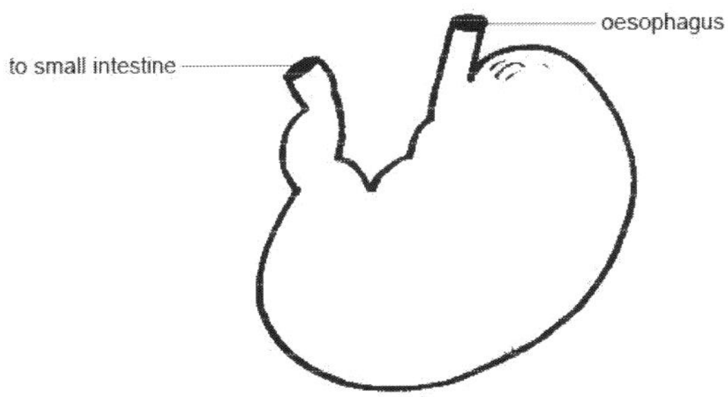

Fig. 11.7-The stomach

SMALL INTESTINE

Most of the breakdown of the large food molecules and absorption of the smaller molecules take place in the long and narrow small intestine. The total length varies but it is about 6.5 metres in humans, 21 metres in the horse, 40 metres in the ox and over 150 metres in the blue whale.

It is divided into 3 sections: the duodenum (after the stomach), jejunum and ileum. The duodenum receives 3 different secretions:

(1) Bile from the liver;

(2) Pancreatic juice from the pancreas and

(3) Intestinal juice from glands in the intestinal wall.

These complete the digestion of starch, fats and protein. The products of digestion are absorbed into the blood and lymphatic system through the wall of the intestine, which is lined with tiny finger-like projections called villi that increase the surface area for more efficient absorption.

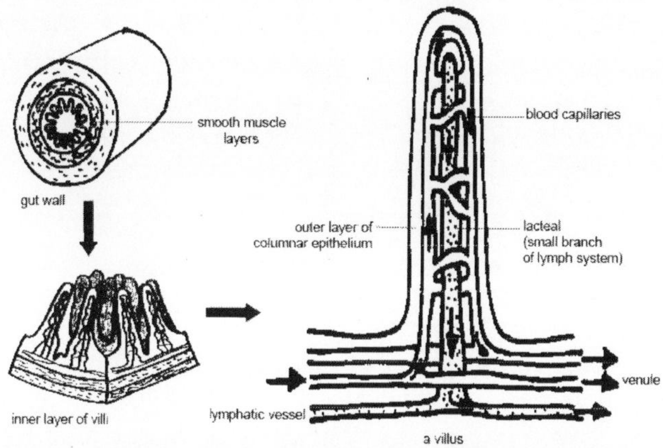

Fig. 11.8 The wall of the small intestine showing villi

THE RUMEN

In ruminant herbivores like cows, sheep and antelopes the stomach is highly modified to act as a "fermentation vat". It is divided into four parts. The largest part is called the rumen . In the cow it occupies the entire left half of the abdominal cavity and can hold up to 270 litres. The reticulum is much smaller and has a honeycomb of raised folds on its inner surface. In the camel the reticulum is further modified to store water. The next part is called the omasum with a folded inner surface. Camels have no omasum. The final compartment is called the abomasum . This is the 'true' stomach where muscular walls churn the food and gastric juice is secreted.

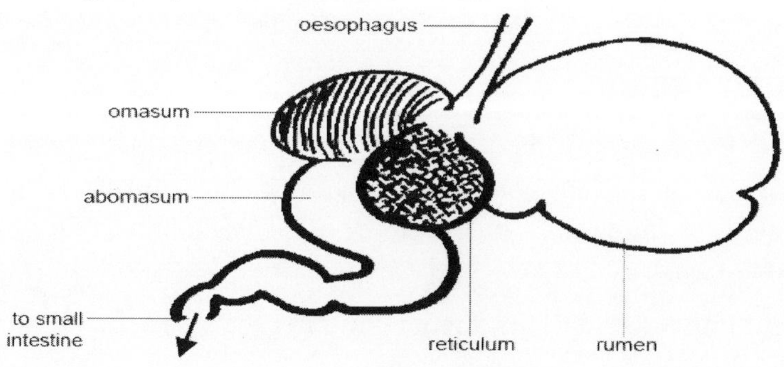

Fig. 11.9 -The rumen

Ruminants swallow the grass they graze almost without chewing and it passes down the oesophagus to the rumen and reticulum. Here liquid is added and the muscular walls churn the food. These chambers provide the main fermentation vat of the ruminant stomach. Here bacteria and single-celled animals start to act on the cellulose plant cell walls. These organisms break down the cellulose to smaller molecules that are absorbed to provide the cow or sheep with energy. In the process, the gases methane and carbon dioxide are produced. These cause the "burps" you may hear cows and sheep making.

Not only do the micro-organisms break down the cellulose but they also produce the vita- mins E, B and K for use by the animal. Their digested bodies provide the ruminant with the majority of its protein requirements.

In the wild grazing is a dangerous activity as it exposes the herbivore to predators. They crop the grass as quickly as possible and then when the animal is in a safer place the food in the rumen can be regurgitated to be chewed at the animal's leisure. This is 'chewing the cud' or rumination. The finely ground food may be returned to the rumen for further work by the microorganisms or, if the particles are small enough, it will pass down a special groove in the wall of the oesophagus straight into the omasum. Here the contents are kneaded and water is absorbed before they pass to the abomasum. The abomasum acts as a "proper" stomach and gastric juice is secreted to digest the protein.

Large Intestine

The large intestine consists of the caecum , colon and rectum . The chyme from the small intestine that enters the colon consists mainly of water and undigested material such as cellulose (fibre or roughage). In omnivores like the pig and humans the main function of

FUNCTIONAL CAECUM

The caecum in the rabbit, rat and guinea pig is greatly enlarged to provide a "fermentation vat" for micro-organisms to break down the cellulose plant cell walls. This is called a functional caecum. In the horse both the caecum and the colon are enlarged. As in the rumen, the large cellulose molecules are broken down to smaller molecules that can be absorbed. However, the position of the functional caecum after the main areas of digestion and absorption, means it is potentially less effective than the rumen. This means that the small molecules that are produced there can not be absorbed by the gut but pass out in the faeces. The rabbit and rodents (and foals) solve this problem by eating their own faeces so that they pass through the gut a second time and the products of cellulose digestion can be absorbed in the small intestine. Rabbits produce two kinds of faeces. Softer night-time faeces are eaten directly from the anus and the harder pellets you are probably familiar with, that have passed through the gut twice.

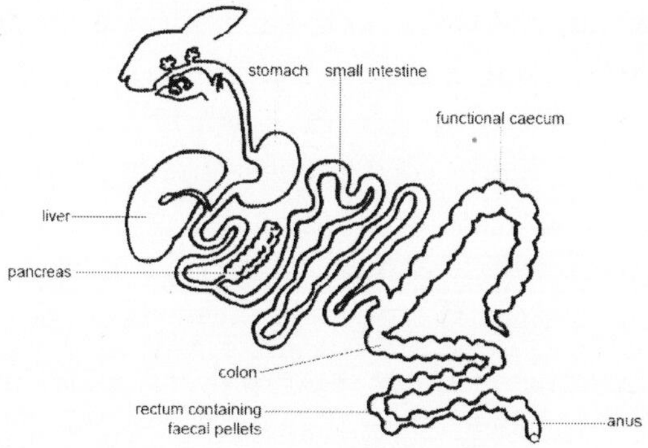

Fig. 11.10 The gut of a rabbit

THE GUT OF BIRDS

Birds' guts have important differences from mammals' guts. Most obviously, birds have a beak instead of teeth. Beaks are much lighter than teeth and are an adaptation for flight. Imagine a bird trying to take off and fly with a whole set of teeth in its head! At the base of the oesophagus birds have a bag-like structure called a crop . In many birds the crop stores food before it enters the stomach, while in pigeons and doves glands in the crop secretes a special fluid called crop-milk which parent birds regurgitate to feed their young. The stomach is also modified and consists of two compartments. The first is the true stomach with muscular walls and enzyme secreting glands. The second compartment is the gizzard.

In seed eating birds this has very muscular walls and contains pebbles swallowed by the bird to help grind the food. This is the reason why you must always supply a caged bird with grit. In birds of prey like the falcon the walls of the gizzard are much thinner and expand to accommodate large meals.

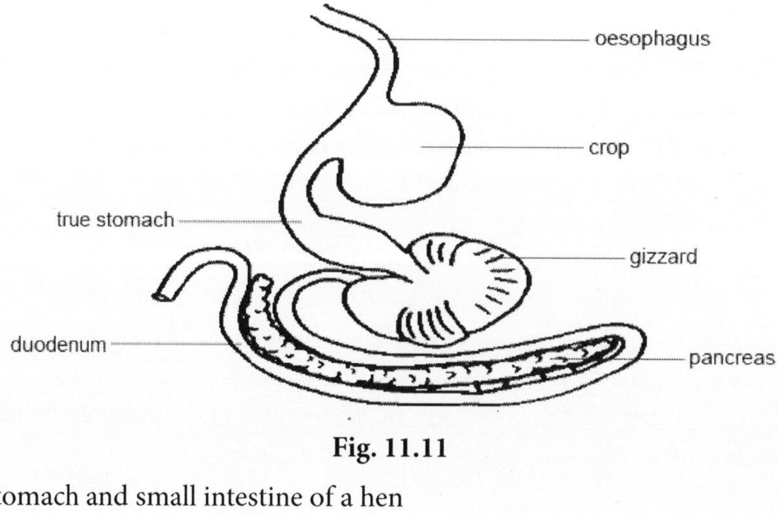

Fig. 11.11

The stomach and small intestine of a hen

Digestion

During digestion the large food molecules are broken down into smaller molecules by en- zymes. The three most important groups of enzymes secreted into the gut are:

1. Amylases that split carbohydrates like starch and glycogen into monosaccharides like glucose.
2. Proteases that split proteins into amino acids.
3. Lipases that split lipids or fats into fatty acids and glycerol.

Glands produce various secretions which mix with the food as it passes along the gut. These secretions include:

1. Saliva secreted into the mouth from several pairs of salivary glands. Saliva consists mainly of water but contains salts, mucous and salivary amy- lase. The function of saliva is to lubricate food as it is chewed and swallowed and salivary amylase begins the digestion of starch.
2. Gastric juice secreted into the stomach from glands in its walls. Gastric juice contains pepsin that breaks down protein and hydrochloric acid to produce the acidic conditions under which this enzyme works best. In baby animals rennin to digest milk is also produced in the stomach.
3. Bile produced by the liver. It is stored in the gall bladder and secreted into the duodenum via the bile duct. (Note that the horse, deer, parrot and rat have no gall bladder). Bile is not a digestive enzyme. Its function is to break up large globules of fat into smaller ones so the fat splitting enzymes can gain access the fat molecules.

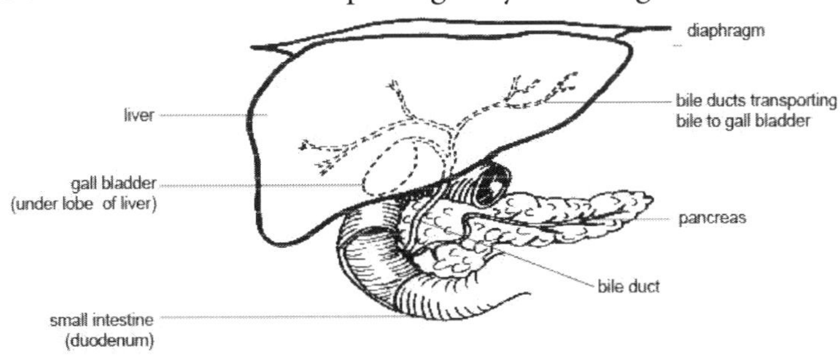

Fig. 11.12

The liver, gall bladder and pancreas

PANCREATIC JUICE

The pancreas is a gland located near the beginning of the duodenum. In most animals it is large and easily seen but in rodents and rabbits it lies within the membrane linking the loops of the intestine (the mesentery) and is quite difficult to find. Pancreatic juice is produced in the pancreas. It flows into the duodenum and contains amylase for digesting starch, lipase for digesting fats and protease for digesting proteins.

INTESTINAL JUICE

Intestinal juice is produced by glands in the lining of the small intestine. It contains enzymes for digesting disaccharides and proteins as well as mucus and salts to make the contents of the small intestine more alkaline so the enzymes can work.

Absorption

The small molecules produced by digestion are absorbed into the villi of the wall of the small intestine . The tiny finger-like projections of the villi increase the surface area for absorption. Glucose and amino acids pass directly through the wall into the blood stream by diffusion or active transport. Fatty acids and glycerol enter vessels of the lymphatic system (lacteals) that run up the centre of each villus.

The Liver

The liver is situated in the abdominal cavity adjacent to the diaphragm (see diagrams 2 and 14). It is the largest single organ of the body and has over 100 known functions. Its most important digestive functions are:

1. the production of bile to help the digestion of fats (described above) and
2. the control of blood sugar levels

Glucose is absorbed into the capillaries of the villi of the intestine. The blood stream takes it directly to the liver via a blood vessel known as the hepatic portal vessel or vein.

The liver converts this glucose into glycogen which it stores. When glucose levels are low the liver can convert the glycogen back into glucose. It releases this back into the blood to keep the level of glucose constant. The hormone insulin , produced by special cells in the pancreas , controls this process.

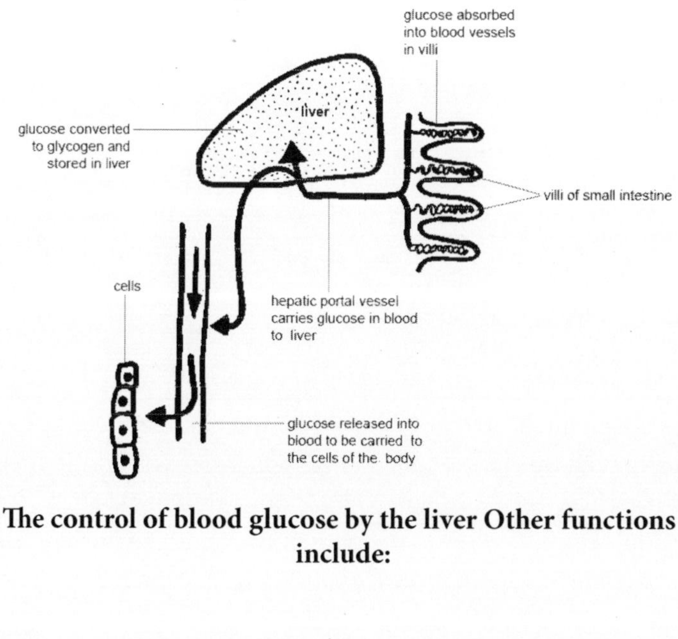

Fig. 11.13 The control of blood glucose by the liver Other functions of the liver include:

3. making vitamin A ,
4. making the proteins that are found in the blood plasma (albumin, globulin and fibrinogen),
5. storing iron ,
6. removing toxic substances like alcohol and poisons from the blood and converting them to safer substances,
7. producing heat to help maintain the temperature of the body.

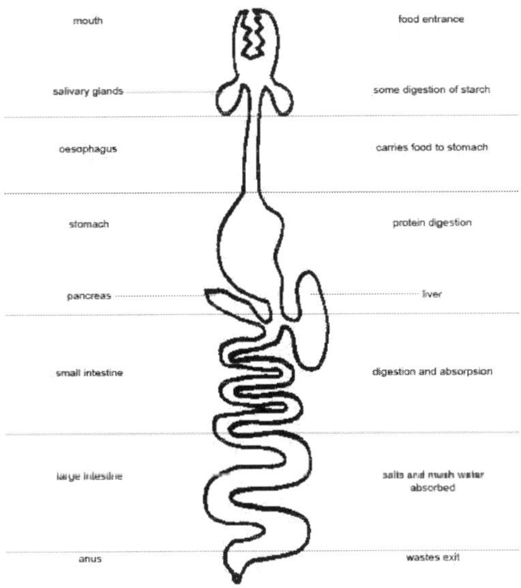

Fig. 11.14

12

URINARY SYSTEM

The cells of an animal can only remain healthy if the conditions are just right. The processes that take place in them are upset if the temperature is too high or too low, or if the fluid around or inside them is too acid or alkaline. Homeostasis is the name given to the processes that help keep the internal conditions constant even when external conditions change. The word means, "staying the same". There are a number of organs in the body that play a part in maintaining homeostasis. For example, the skin helps keep the internal temperature of bird and mammals bodies within a narrow range even when the outside temperatures change; the lungs control the amount of carbon dioxide in the blood; the liver and pancreas work together to keep the amount of glucose in the blood within narrow limits and the kidneys regulate the acidity and the concentration of water and salt in the blood. How the kidneys do this will be described later in this chapter.

Hormones are chemicals that carry messages around the body in the blood and are central to many of the homeostatic processes mentioned above.

WATER IN THE BODY

Water is essential for living things to survive because all the chemical reactions within a body take place in a solution of water. An animal's body consists of up to 80% water. The exact proportion depends on the type of animal, its age, sex, health and whether or not it has had sufficient to drink. Generally animals do not survive a loss of more than 15% of their body water.

Maintaining Water Balance

In vertebrates almost 2/3rd of this water is in the cells (intracellular fluid). The rest is outside the cells (extracellular fluid) where it is found in the spaces around the cells (tissue fluid), as well as in the blood and lymph.

Maintaining Water Balance

Animals lose water through their skin and lungs, in the faeces and urine. These losses must be made up by water in food and drink and from the water that is a by-product of chemical reactions. If the animal does not manage to compensate for water loss the dissolved substances in the blood may become so concentrated they become lethal. To prevent this happening various mechanisms come into play as soon as the concentration of the blood increases. A part of the brain called the hypothalamus is in charge of these homeostatic processes. The most important is the feeling of thirst that is triggered by an increase in blood concentration. This stimulates an animal to find water and drink it.

The kidneys are also involved in maintaining water balance as various hormones instruct them to produce more concentrated urine and so retain some of the water that would otherwise be lost.

DESERT ANIMALS

Coping with water loss is a particular problem for animals that live in dry conditions. Some, like the camel, have developed great tolerance for dehydration. For example, under some conditions, camels can withstand the loss of one third of their body mass as water. They can also survive wide daily changes in temperature. This means they do not have to use large quantities of water in sweat to cool the body by evaporation.

Smaller animals are more able than large ones to avoid extremes of temperature or dry conditions by resting in sheltered more humid situations during the day and being active only at night.

The kangaroo rat is able to survive without access to any drinking water at all because it does not sweat and produces extremely concentrated urine. Water from its food and from chemical processes is sufficient to supply all its requirements.

Excretion

Animals need to excrete because they take in substances that are excess to the body's requirements and many of the chemical reactions in the body produce waste products. If these substances were not removed they would poison cells or slow down metabolism. All animals therefore have some means of getting rid of these wastes.

The major waste products in mammals are carbon dioxide that is removed by the lungs, and urea that is produced when excess amino acids (from proteins) are broken down. Urea is filtered from the blood by the kidneys.

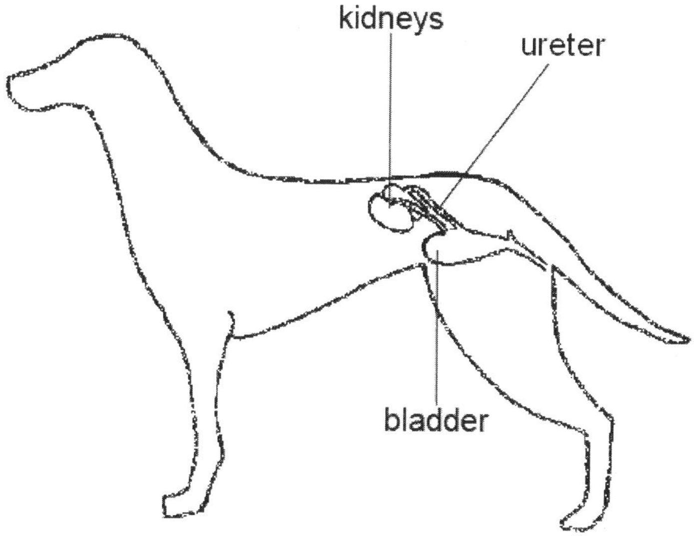

Fig. 12.1 The position of the organs of the urinary system in a dog

THE KIDNEYS AND URINARY SYSTEM

The kidneys in mammals are bean-shaped organs that lie in the abdominal cavity attached to the dorsal wall on either side of the spine. An artery from the dorsal aorta called the renal artery supplies blood to them and the renal vein drains them.

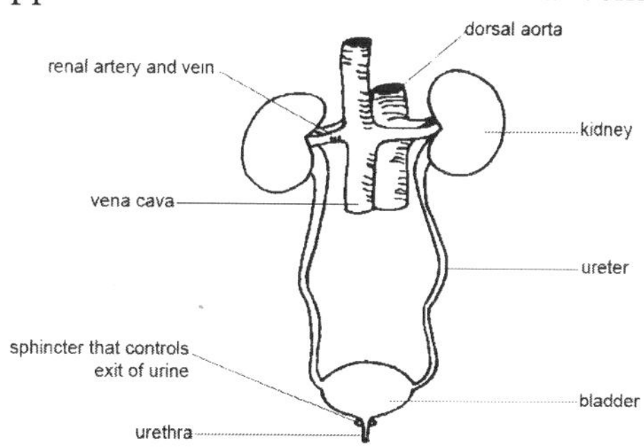

Fig. 12.2

The urinary system

To the naked eye kidneys seem simple enough organs. They are covered by a fibrous coat or capsule and if cut in half lengthways (longitudinally) two distinct regions can be seen - an inner region or medulla and the outer cortex. A cavity within the kidney called the pelvis collects the urine and carries it to the ureter, which connects with the bladder where the urine is stored temporarily. Rings of muscle (sphincters) control the release of urine from the bladder and the urine leaves the body through the urethra.

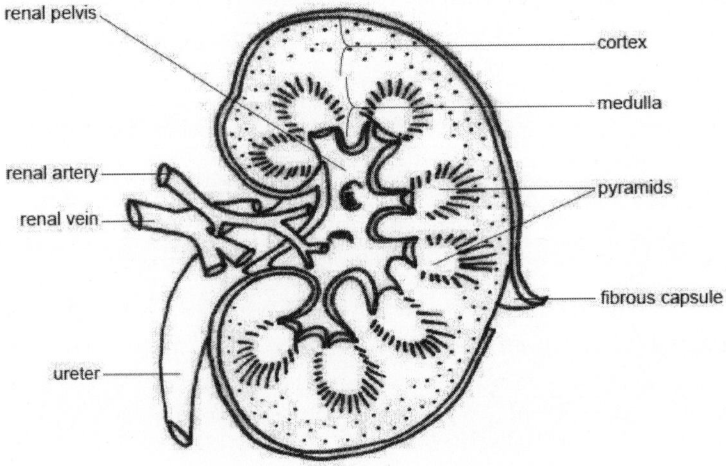

Fig. 12.3 The dissected kidney

KIDNEY TUBULES OR NEPHRONS

It is only when you examine kidneys under the microscope that you find that their structure is not simple at all. The cortex and medulla are seen to be composed of masses of tiny tubes. These are called kidney tubules or nephrons. A human kidney consists of over a million of them.

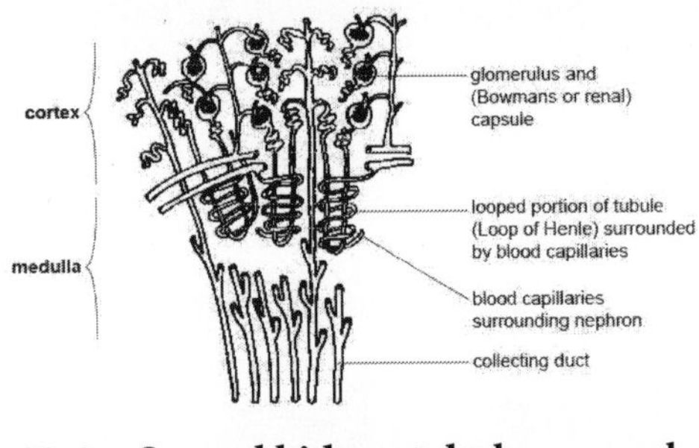

Fig. 12.4 a Several kidney tubules or nephrons

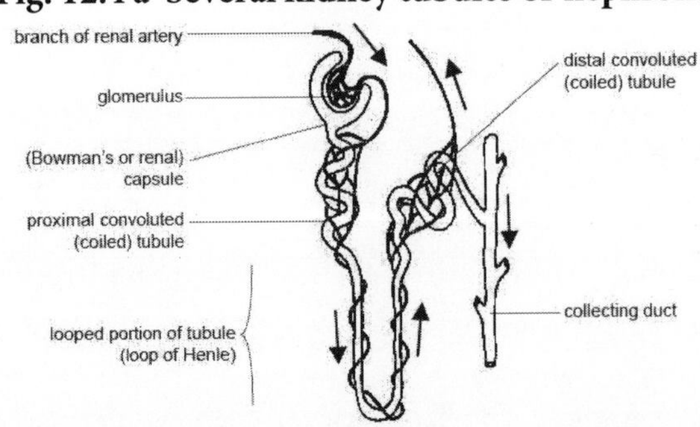

Fig. 12.4 b - A kidney tubule or nephron

At one end of each nephron, in the cortex of the kidney, is a cup shaped structure called the (Bowman's or renal) capsule. It surrounds a tuft of capillaries called the glomerulus that carries high-pressure blood. Together the glomerulus and capsule act as a blood-filtering device. The holes in the filter allow most of the contents of the blood through except the red and white cells and large protein molecules. The fluid flowing from the capsule into the rest of the kidney tubule is therefore very similar to blood plasma and contains many useful substances like water, glucose, salt and amino acids. It also contains waste products like urea .

PROCESSES OCCURRING IN THE NEPHRON

After entering the glomerulus the filtered fluid flows along a coiled part of the tubule (the proximal convoluted tubule) to a looped portion (the Loop of Henle) and then to the collecting tube via a second length of coiled tube (the distal convoluted tubule.

From the collecting ducts the urine flows into the renal pelvis and enters the ureter .

Note that the glomerulus, capsule and both coiled parts of the tubule are all situated in the cortex of the kidney while the loops of Henle and collecting ducts make up the medulla.

As the fluid flows along the proximal convoluted tubule useful substances like glucose, water, salts, potassium ions, calcium ions and amino acids are reabsorbed into the blood capil- laries that form a network around the tubules. Many of these substances are transported by active transport and energy is required.

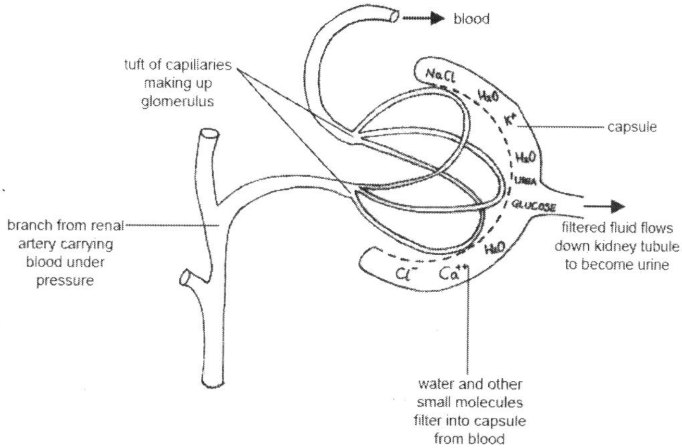

Fig. 12.5 Filtration in the glomerulus and capsule

In a separate process, some substances, particularly potassium, ammonium and hydrogen ions, and drugs like penicillin, are actively secreted into the distal convoluted tubule.

By the time the fluid has reached the collecting ducts these processes of absorption and secretion have changed the fluid originally filtered into the Bowman's capsule into urine. The main function of the collecting ducts is then to remove more water from the urine if necessary.

Normal urine consists of water, in which waste products such as urea and salts such as sodium chloride are dissolved. Pigments from the breakdown of red blood cells give urine its yellow colour.

THE PRODUCTION OF CONCENTRATED URINE

Because of the high pressure of the blood in the glomerulus and the large size of the pores in the glomerulus/capsule-filtering device, an enormous volume of fluid passes into the kidney tubules. If this fluid were left as it is, the animal's body would be drained dry in 30 minutes. In fact, as the fluid flows down the tubule, over 90% of the water in it is reabsorbed. The main part of this reabsorption takes place in the collecting tubes.

The amount of water removed from the collecting ducts is controlled by a hormone called antidiuretic hormone (ADH) produced by the pituitary gland , situated at the base of the brain. When the blood becomes more concentrated, as happens when an animal is deprived of water, ADH is secreted and causes more water to be absorbed from the collecting ducts so that concentrated urine is produced. When the animal has drunk plenty of water and the blood is dilute, no ADH is secreted and no or little water is absorbed from the collecting ducts, so dilute urine is produced. In this way the concentration of the blood is controlled precisely.

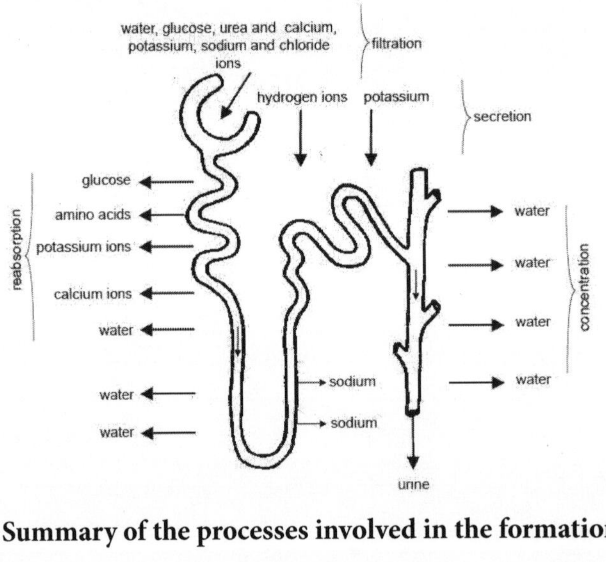

Fig. 12.6 Summary of the processes involved in the formation of urine

WATER BALANCE IN FISH AND MARINE ANIMALS

Fresh Water Fish

Although the skin of fish is more or less waterproof, the gills are very porous. The body fluids of fish that live in fresh water have a higher concentration of dissolved substances than the water in which they swim. In other words the body fluids of fresh water fish are hypertonic to the water. Water therefore flows into the body by osmosis

To stop the body fluids being constantly diluted fresh water fish produce large quantities of dilute urine.

Marine Fish

Marine fish like the sharks and dogfish have body fluids that have the same concentration of dissolved substances as the water (isotonic) have little problem with water balance. However, marine bony fish like red cod, snapper and sole, have body fluids with a lower concentration of dissolved substances than seawater (they are hypotonic to seawater). This means that water tends to flow out of their bodies by osmosis. To make up this fluid loss they drink seawater and get rid of the excess salt by excreting it from the gills.

MARINE BIRDS

Marine birds that eat marine fish take in large quantities of salt and some only have access to seawater for drinking. Bird's kidneys are unable to produce very concentrated urine, so they have developed a salt gland. This excretes a concentrated salt solution into the nose to get rid of the excess salt.

Diabetes And The Kidney

There are two types of diabetes. The most common is called sugar diabetes or diabetes mellitus and is common in cats and dogs especially if they are overweight. It is caused by the pancreas secreting insufficient insulin , the hormone that controls the amount of glucose in the blood. If insulin secretion is inadequate, the concentration of glucose in the blood increases. Any increase in the glucose in the blood automatically leads to an increase in glucose in the fluid filtered into the kidney tubule. Normally the kidney removes all the glucose filtered into it, but these high concentrations swamp this removal mechanism and urine containing glucose is produced. The main symptoms of this type of diabetes are the production of large amounts of dilute urine containing glucose, and excessive thirst.

The second type of diabetes is called diabetes insipidus . The name comes from the main symptom, which is the production of large amounts of very dilute and "tasteless" urine. It occurs when the pituitary gland produces insufficient ADH, the hormone that stimulates water re-absorption from the kidney tubule. When this hormone is lacking, water is not absorbed and large amounts of dilute urine are produced. Because so much water is lost in the urine, animals with this form of diabetes can die if deprived of water for only a day or so.

OTHER FUNCTIONS OF THE KIDNEY

The excretion of urea from the body and the maintenance of water balance, as described above, are the main functions of the kidney. However, the kidneys have other roles in keeping conditions in the body stable i.e. in maintaining homeostasis. These include:

- controlling the concentration of salt ions (Na+, K+, Cl-) in the blood by adjusting how much is excreted or retained;
- maintaining the correct acidity of the blood. Excess acid is constantly being produced by the normal chemical reactions in the body and the kidney eliminates this.

NORMAL URINE

Normal Urine

Normal urine consists of water (95%), urea, salts (mostly sodium chloride) and pigments (mostly from bile) that give it its characteristic colour.

Abnormal Ingredients Of Urine

If the body is not working properly, small amounts of substances not normally present may be found in the urine or substances normally present may appear in abnormal amounts.

- The presence of glucose may indicate diabetes (see above).
- Urine with red blood cells in it is called haematuria , and may indicate inflammation of the kidney,or urinary tract, cancer or a blow to the kidneys.
- Sometimes free haemoglobin is found in the urine. This indicates that the red blood cells in the blood have haemolysed (the membrane has broken down) and the haemoglobin has passed into the kidney tubules.
- The presence of white blood cells in the urine indicates there is an infection in the kidney or urinary tract.
- Protein molecules are usually too large to pass into the kidney tubule so no or only small amounts of proteins like albumin is normally found in urine. Large quantities of albumin indicate that the kidney tubules have been injured or the kidney has become diseased. High blood pressure also pushes proteins from the blood into the tubules.
- Casts are tiny cylinders of material that have been shed from the lining of the tubules and flushed out into the urine.
- Mucus is not usually found in the urine of healthy animals but is a normal constituent of horses' urine, giving it a characteristic cloudy appearance.

Tests can be carried out to identify any abnormal ingredients of urine. These tests are normally done by "stix ", which are small plastic strips with absorbent ends impregnated with various chemicals. A colour change occurs in the presence of an abnormal ingredient.

EXCRETION IN BIRDS

Birds' high body temperature and level of activity means that they need to conserve water. Birds therefore do not have a bladder and instead of excreting urea, which needs to be dissolved in large amounts of water, birds produce uric acid that can be discharged as a thick paste along with the feces. This is the white chalky part of the bird droppings that land on you or your car.

13

NERVOUS SYSTEM

Animals must be able to sense and respond to the environment in which they live if they are to survive. They need to be able to sense the temperature of their surroundings, for example, so they can avoid the hot sun. They must also be able to identify food and escape predators.

The various systems and organs in the body must also be linked so they work together. For example, once a predator has identified suitable prey it has to catch it. This involves coordinating the contraction of the muscle so the predator can run, there must then be an increased blood supply to the muscles to provide them with oxygen and nutrients. At the same time the respiration rate must increase to supply the oxygen and remove the carbon dioxide produced as a result of this increased activity. Once the prey has been caught and eaten, the digestive system must be activated to digest it.

The adjustment of an animal's response to changes in the environment and the complex linking of the various processes in the body that this response involves are called co-ordination.

Two systems are involved in co-ordination in animals. These are the nervous and endocrine systems. The first operates via electrical impulses along nerve fibres and the second by releasing special chemicals or hormones into the bloodstream from glands.

FUNCTIONS OF THE NERVOUS SYSTEM

The nervous system has three basic functions:

1. Sensory function - to sense changes (known as stimuli) both outside and within the body. For example the eyes sense changes in light and the ear responds to sound waves.

Inside the body, stretch receptors in the stomach indicate when it is full and chemical receptors in the blood vessels monitor the acidity of the blood.

2. Integrative function - processing the information received from the sense organs. The impulses from these organs are analysed and stored as memory. The many different impulses from different sources are sorted, synchronised and co-ordinated and the appro- priate response initiated. The power to integrate, remember and apply experience gives higher animals much of their superiority.

3. Motor function - The third function is the response to the stimuli that causes muscles to contract or glands to secrete.

All nervous tissue is made up of nerve cells or neurons. These transmit high-speed signals called nerve impulses . Nerve impulses can be thought of as being similar to an electric current.

The Neuron

Neurons are cells that have been adapted to carry nerve impulses. A typical neuron has a cell body containing a nucleus, one or more branching filaments called dendrites which conduct nerve impulses towards the cell body and one long fibre, an axon , that carries the impulses away from it. Many axons have a sheath of fatty material called myelin surrounding them. This speeds up the rate at which the nerve impulses travel along the nerve.

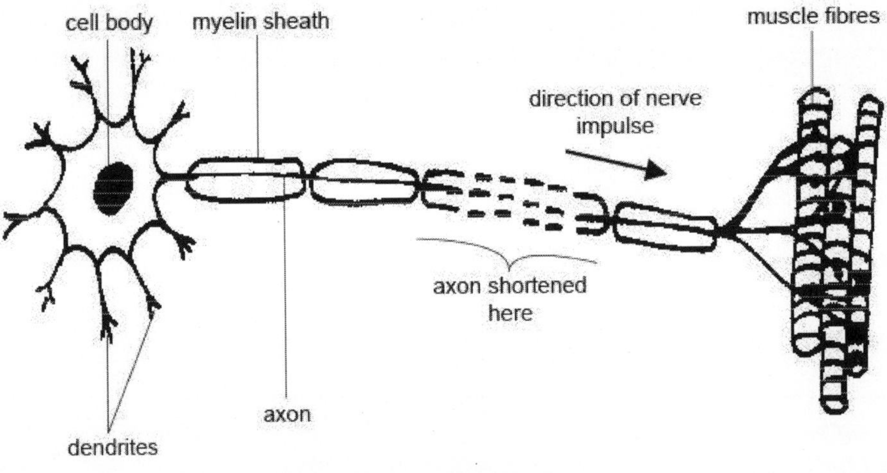

Fig. 13.1 A motor neuron

The cell body of neurons is usually located in the brain or spinal cord while the axon extends the whole distance to the organ that it supplies. The neuron carrying impulses from the spinal cord to the hind leg or tail of a horse, for example, can be several feet long. A nerve is a bundle of axons.

A sensory neuron is a nerve cell that transmits impulses from a sense receptor such as those in the eye or ear to the brain or spinal cord. A motor neuron is a nerve cell that transmits impulses from the brain or spinal cord to a muscle or gland. A relay neuron connects sensory and motor neurons and is found in the brain or spinal cord.

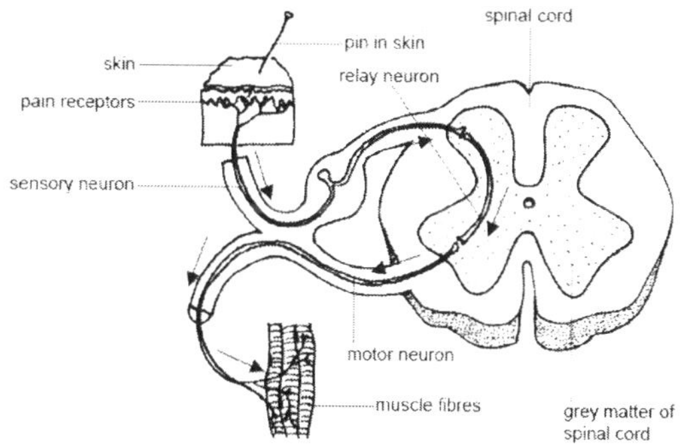

Fig. 13.2

CONNECTIONS BETWEEN NEURONS

The connection between adjacent neurons is called a synapse . The two nerve cells do not actually touch here for there is a microscopic space between them. The electrical impulse in the neurone before the synapse stimulates the production of chemicals called neurotransmitters (such as acetylcholine), which are secreted into the gap.

The neurotransmitter chemicals diffuse across the gap and when they contact the membrane of the next nerve cell they stimulate a new nervous impulse. After the impulse has passed the chemical is destroyed and the synapse is ready to receive the next nerve impulse.

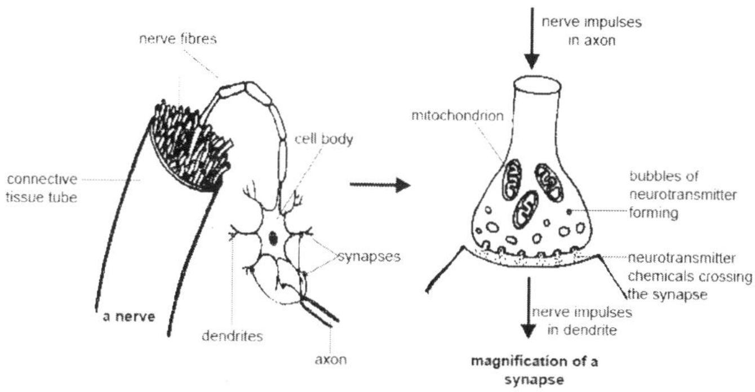

Fig. 13.3

Reflexes

A reflex is a rapid automatic response to a stimulus. When you accidentally touch a hot object and automatically jerk your hand away, this is a reflex action. It happens without you having to think about it. Animals automatically blink when an object approaches the eye and cats twist their bodies in the air when falling so they land on their paws. (Please don't test this one at home with your pet cat!).

Swallowing, sneezing, and the constriction of the pupil of the eye in bright light are also all reflex actions.

The path taken by the nerve impulses in a reflex is called a reflex arc . Most reflex arcs involve only three neurons. The stimulus (a pin in the paw) stimulates the pain receptors of the skin, which initiate an impulse in a sensory neuron. This travels to the spinal cord where it passes, by means of a synapse, to a connecting neuron called the relay neuron situated in the spinal cord. The relay neuron in turn makes a synapse with one or more motor neurons that transmit the impulse to the muscles of the limb causing them to contract and remove the paw from the sharp object. Reflexes do not require involvement of the brain although you are aware of what is happening and can, in some instances, prevent them happening. Animals are born with their reflexes. You can think of them as being wired in.

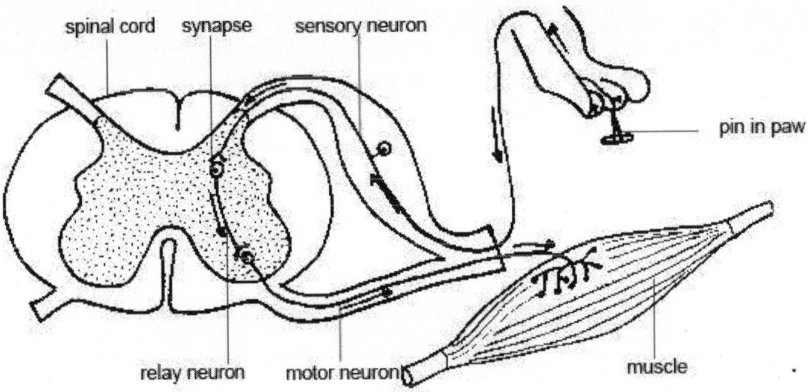

Fig. 13.4

CONDITIONED REflEXES

In most reflexes the stimulus and response are related. For example the presence of food in the mouth causes the salivary glands to release saliva. However, it is possible to train animals (and humans) to respond to different and often quite irrelevant stimuli. This is called a conditioned reflex .

A Russian biologist called Pavlov carried out the classic experiment to demonstrate such a reflex when he conditioned dogs to salivate at the sound of a bell ringing. Almost every pet owner can identify reflexes they have conditioned in their animals. Perhaps you have trained your cat to associate food with the opening of the fridge door or accustomed your dog to the routines you go through before taking them for a walk.

Parts of the Nervous System

When we describe the nervous system of vertebrates we usually divide it into two parts.

1. The central nervous system (CNS) which consists of the brain and spinal cord.

2. The peripheral nervous system (PNS) which consists of the nerves that connect to the brain and spinal cord (cranial and spinal nerves) as well as the autonomic (or involuntary) nervous system.

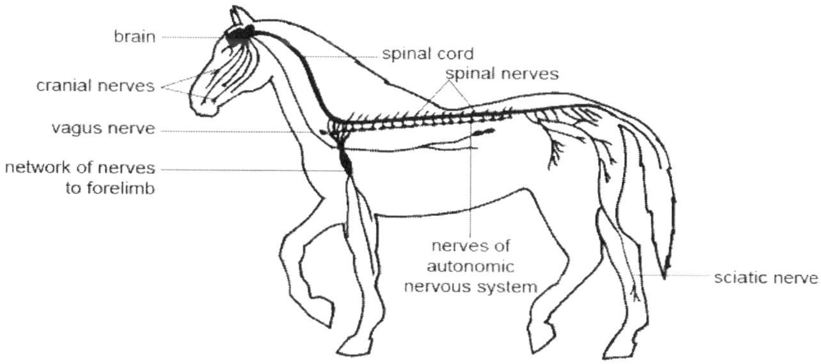

Fig. 13.5

Diagram 13.5 - The nervous system of a horse

The Central Nervous System

The central nervous system consists of the brain and spinal cord. It acts as a kind of 'telephone exchange' where a vast number of cross connections are made.

When you look at the brain or spinal cord some regions appear creamy white (white matter) and others appear grey (grey matter). White matter consists of masses of nerve axons and the grey matter consists of the nerve cells. In the brain the grey matter is on the outside and in the spinal cord it is on the inside .

The Brain

The major part of the brain lies protected within the sturdy "box" of skull called the cranium . Surrounding the fragile brain tissue (and spinal cord) are protective membranes called the meninges, and a crystal-clear fluid called cerebrospinal fluid , which protects and nourishes the brain tissue. This fluid also fills four cavities or ventricles that lie within the brain.

Brain tissue is extremely active and, even when an animal is resting, it uses up to 20% of the oxygen taken into the body by the lungs. The carotid artery , a branch off the dorsal aorta, supplies it with the oxygen and nutrients it requires. Brain damage occurs if brain tissue is deprived of oxygen for only 4-8 minutes.

The brain consists of three major regions:

1. the fore brain which includes the cerebral hemispheres , hypothalamus and pituitary gland ;
2. the hind brain or brain stem , contains the medulla oblongata and pons and
3. the cerebellum or "little brain".

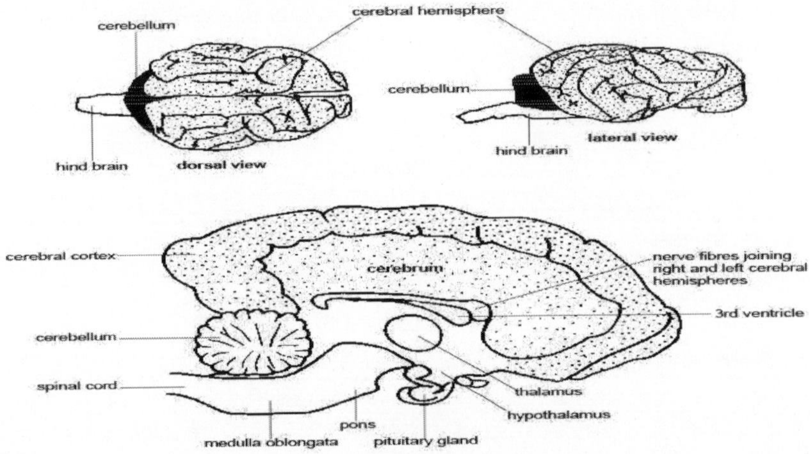

Fig. 13.6

Diagram 13.6 - Longitudinal section through the brain of a dog

MAPPING THE BRAIN

In humans and some animals the functions of the different regions of the cerebral cortex have been mapped.

The Forebrain

The cerebral hemispheres are the masses of brain tissue that sit on the top of the brain. The surface is folded into ridges and furrows called sulci (singular sulcus). They make this part of the brain look rather like a very large walnut kernel. The two hemispheres are separated by a deep groove although they are connected internally by a thick bundle of nerve fibres. The outer layer of each hemisphere is called the cerebral cortex and this is where the main functions of the cerebral hemispheres are carried out.

The cerebral cortex is large and convoluted in mammals compared to other vertebrates and largest of all in humans because this is where the so-called "higher centres" concerned with memory, learning, reasoning and intelligence are situated.

Nerves from the eyes, ears, nose and skin bring sensory impulses to the cortex where they are interpreted. Appropriate voluntary movements are initiated here in the light of the memories of past events.

Different regions of the cortex are responsible for particular sensory and motor functions, e.g. vision, hearing, taste, smell, or moving the fore-limbs, hind-limbs or tail. For example, when a dog sniffs a scent, sensory impulses from the organ of smell in the nose pass via the olfactory (smelling) nerve to the olfactory centres of the cerebral hemispheres where the impulses are interpreted and co-ordinated.

In humans and some animals the functions of the different regions of the cerebral cortex have been mapped.

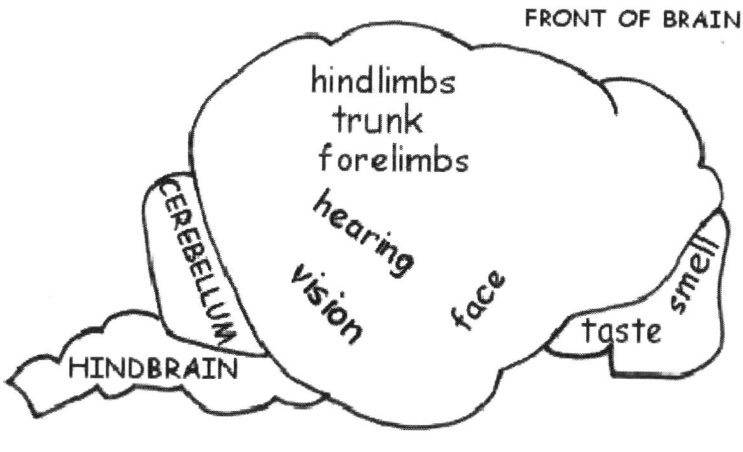

Fig. 13.7

The hypothalamus is situated at the base of the brain and is connected by a "stalk" to the pituitary gland , the "master" hormone-producing gland. The hypothalamus can be thought of as the bridge between the nervous and endocrine (hormone producing) systems. It produces some of the hormones that are released from the pituitary gland and controls the release of others from it.

It is also an important centre for controlling the internal environment of the animal and therefore maintaining homeostasis. For example, it helps regulate the movement of food through the gut and the temperature, blood pressure and concentration of the blood. It is also responsible for the feeling of being hungry or thirsty and it controls sleep patterns and sex drive.

The Hindbrain

The medulla oblongata is at the base of the brain and is a continuation of the spinal cord. It carries all signals between the spinal cord and the brain and contains centres that control vital body functions like the basic rhythm of breathing, the rate of the heartbeat and the activities of the gut. The medulla oblongata also co-ordinates swallowing, vomiting, coughing and sneezing.

The Cerebellum

The cerebellum (little brain) looks rather like a smaller version of the cerebral hemispheres attached to the back of the brain. It receives impulses from the organ of balance (vestibular organ) in the inner ear and from stretch receptors in the muscles and tendons. By co- ordinating these it regulates muscle contraction during walking and running and helps maintain the posture and balance of the animal. When the cerebellum malfunctions it causes a tremor and uncoordinated movement.

The Spinal Cord

The spinal cord is a cable of nerve tissue that passes down the channel in the vertebrae from the hindbrain to the end of the tail. It becomes progressively smaller as paired spinal nerves pass out of the cord to parts of the body. Protective membranes or meninges cover the cord and these enclose cerebral spinal fluid.

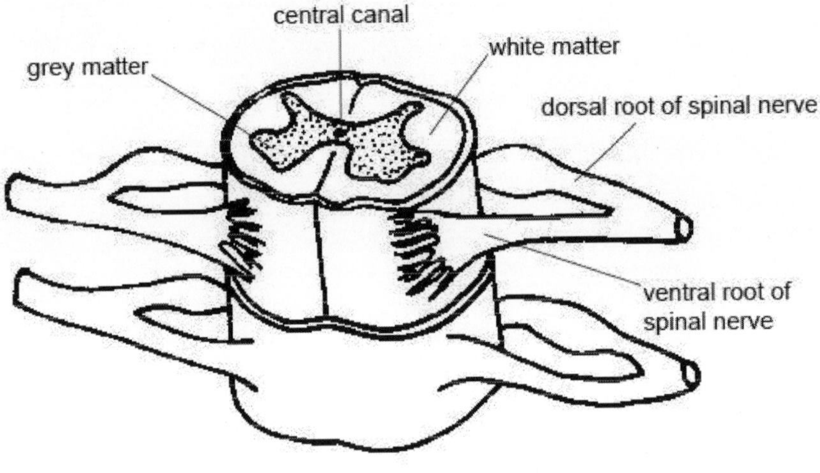

Fig. 13.8

If you cut across the spinal cord you can see that it consists of white matter on the outside and grey matter in the shape of an H or butterfly on the inside.

THE PERIPHERAL NERVOUS SYSTEM

The peripheral nervous system consists of nerves that are connected to the brain (cranial nerves), and nerves that are connected to the spinal cord (spinal nerves). The autonomic nervous system is also part of the peripheral nervous system.

Cranial Nerves

There are twelve pairs of cranial nerves that come from the brain. Each passes through a hole in the cranium (brain case). The most important of these are the olfactory, optic, acoustic and vagus nerves.

The olfactory nerves - (smell) carry impulses from the olfactory organ of the nose to the brain.

The optic nerves - (sight) carry impulses from the retina of the eye to the brain.

The auditory (acoustic) nerves - (hearing) carry impulses from the cochlear of the inner ear to the brain.

The vagus nerve - controls the muscles that bring about swallowing. It also controls the muscles of the heart, airways, lungs, stomach and intestines.

Spinal Nerves

Spinal nerves connect the spinal cord to sense organs, muscles and glands in the body. Pairs of spinal nerves leave the spinal cord and emerge between each pair of adjacent vertebrae.

The sciatic nerve is the largest spinal nerve in the body. It leaves the spinal cord as several nerves that join to form a flat band of nervous tissue. It passes down the thigh towards the hind leg where it gives off branches to the various muscles of this limb.

THE AUTONOMIC NERVOUS SYSTEM

The autonomic nervous system controls internal body functions that are not under conscious control. For example when a prey animal is chased by a predator the autonomic nervous system automatically increases the rate of breathing and the heartbeat. It dilates the blood vessels that carry blood to the muscles, releases glucose from the liver, and makes other adjustments to provide for the sudden increase in activity. When the animal has escaped and is safe once again the nervous system slows down all these processes and resumes all the normal body activities like the digestion of food.

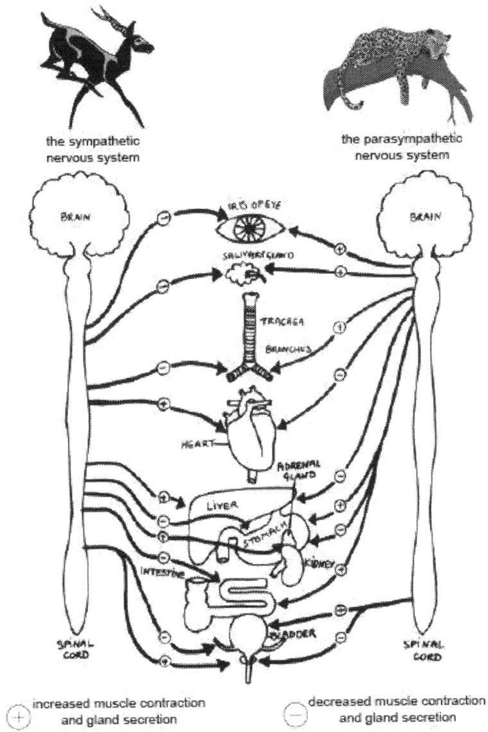

Fig. 13.9

Diagram 13.9 - The function of the sympathetic and parasympathetic nervous systems

The nerves of the autonomic nervous system originate in the spinal cord and pass out between the vertebrae to serve the various organs. There are two main parts to the autonomic nervous system -- the sympathetic system and the parasympathetic system .

The sympathetic system stimulates the "flight, fright, fight" response that allows an animal to face up to an attacker or make a rapid departure. It increases the heart and respiratory rates, as well as the amount of blood flowing to the skeletal muscles while blood flow to less critical regions like the gut and skin is reduced. It also causes the pupils of the eyes to dilate. Note that the effects of the sympathetic system are similar to the effects of the hormone adrenaline.

The parasympathetic system does the opposite to the sympathetic system. It maintains the normal functions of the relaxed body. These are sometimes known as the "housekeeping" functions. It promotes effective digestion, stimulates defaecation and urination and maintains a regular heartbeat and rate of breathing.

Summary

- The neuron is the basic unit of the nervous system. It consists of a cell body with a nucleus, filaments known as dendrites and a long fibre known as the axon often surrounded by a myelin sheath .
- A nerve is a bundle of axons.
- Grey matter in the brain and spinal cord consists mainly of brain cells while white matte r consists of masses of axons.
- Nerve Impulses travel along axons.
- Adjacent neurons connect with each other at synapses .
- Reflexes are automatic responses to stimuli. The path taken by nerve impulses involved in reflexes is a reflex arc . Most reflex arcs involve 3 neurons - a sensory neuron , a relay neuron and a motor neuron . A stimulus, a pin in the paw for example, initiates an impulse in the sensory neuron that passes via a synapse to the relay neuron situated in the spinal cord and then via another synapse to the motor neurone. This transmits the impulse to the muscle causing it to contract and remove the paw from the pin.
- The nervous system is divided into 2 parts: the central nervous system , consisting of the brain and spinal cord and the peripheral nervous system consisting of nerves connected to the brain and spinal cord. The autonomic nervous system is considered to be part of the peripheral nervous system.
- The brain consists of three major regions: 1. the fore brain which includes the cere- bral hemispheres (or cerebrum), hypothalamus and pituitary gland ; 2. the hindbrain or brain stem containing the medulla oblongata and 3. the cerebellum

- Protective membranes known as the meninges surround the brain and spinal cord.
- There are 12 pairs of cranial nerves that include the optic, olfactory, acoustic and vagus

nerves.

- The spinal cord is a cable of nerve tissue surrounded by meninges passing from the brain to the end of the tail. Spinal nerves emerge by a ventral and dorsal root between each vertebra and connect the spinal cord with organs and muscles.
- The autonomic nervous system controls internal body functions not under conscious control. It is divided into 2 parts with 2 different functions: the sympathetic nervous system that is involved in the flight and fight response including increased heart rate, bronchial dilation, dilation of the pupil and decreased gut activity. The parasympa- thetic nervous system is associated with decreased heart rate, pupil constriction and increased gut activity.

14

THE SENSES

Sense organs allow animals to sense changes in the environment around them and in their bodies so that they can respond appropriately. They enable animals to avoid hostile environments, sense the presence of predators and find food.

Animals can sense a wide range of stimuli that includes, touch, pressure, pain, temperature, chemicals, light, sound, movement and position of the body. Some animals can sense electric and magnetic fields. All sense organs respond to stimuli by producing nerve impulses that travel to the brain via a sensory nerve. The impulses are then processed and interpreted in the brain as pain, sight, sound, taste etc.

The senses are often divided into two groups:

3. The general senses of touch, pressure, pain and temperature that are distributed fairly evenly through the skin. Some are found in muscles and within joints.
4. The special senses which include the senses of smell, taste, sight, hearing and balance. The special sense organs may be quite complex in structure.

TOUCH AND PRESSURE

Within the dermis of the skin are numerous modified nerve endings that are sensitive to touch and pressure. The roots of hairs may also be well supplied with sensory receptors that inform the animal that it is in contact with an object. Whiskers are specially modified hairs.

Pain

Receptors that sense pain are found in almost every tissue of the body. They tell the animal that tissues are dangerously hot, cold, compressed or stretched or that there is not enough blood flowing in them. The animal may then be able to respond and protect itself from further damage.

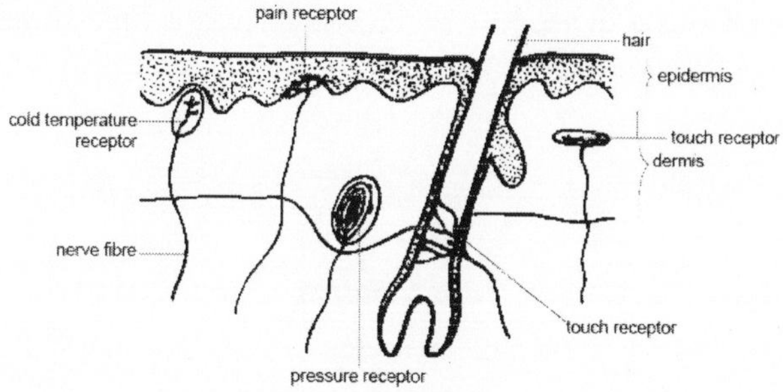

Fig. 14.1

TEMPERATURE

Nerve endings in the skin respond to hot and cold stimuli.

Awareness of Limb Position

There are sense organs in the muscles, tendons and joints that send continuous impulses to the brain that tell it where each limb is. This information allows the animal to place its limbs accurately and know their exact position without having to watch them.

Smell

Animals use the sense of smell to locate food, mark territory, identify their own offspring and the presence and sexual condition of a potential mate. The organ of smell (olfactory organ) is located in the nose and responds to chemicals in the air. It consists of modified nerve cells that have several tiny hairs on the surface. These emerge from the epithelium on

the roof of the nose cavity into the mucus that lines it. As the animal breathes, chemicals in the air dissolve in the mucus. When the sense cell responds to a particular molecule, it fires an impulse that travels along the olfactory nerve to the brain where it is interpreted as an odour.

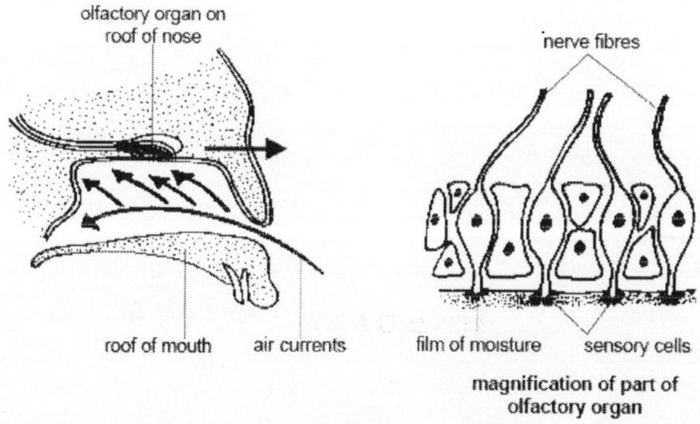

Fig. 14.2

The olfactory sense in humans is rudimentary compared to that of many animals. Carnivores that hunt have a very highly developed sensitivity to scents. For example a polar bear can smell out a dead seal 20 km away and a bloodhound can distinguish between the trails of different people although it may sometimes be confused by the criss-crossing trail of identical twins.

Snakes and lizards detect odours by means of Jacobson's organ . This is situated on the roof of the mouth and consists of pits containing sensory cells. When snakes flick out their forked tongues they are smelling the air by carrying the molecules in it to the Jacobson's organ.

Taste

The sense of taste allows animals to detect and identify dissolved chemicals. In reptiles, birds, and mammals the taste receptors (taste buds) are found mainly to the upper surface of the tongue. They consist of pits containing sensory cells arranged rather like the segments of an orange. Each receptor cell has a tiny "hair" that projects into the saliva to sense the chemicals dissolved in it.

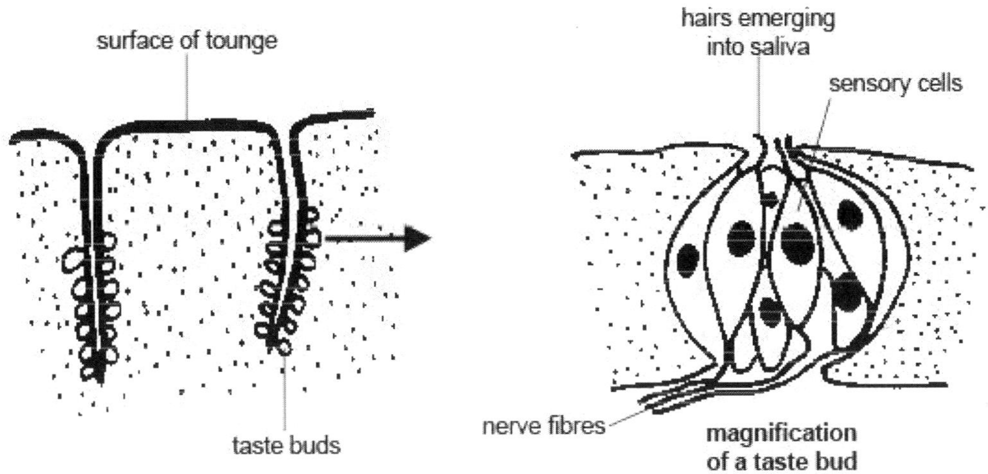

Fig. 14.3

The sense of taste is quite restricted. Humans can only distinguish four different tastes (sweet, sour, bitter and salt) and what we normally think of as taste is mainly the sense of smell. Food is quite tasteless when the nose is blocked and cats often refuse to eat when this happens.

Sight

The eyes are the organs of sight. They consist of spherical eyeballs situated in deep depressions in the skull called the orbits . They are attached to the wall of the orbit by six muscles, which move the eyeball. Upper and lower eyelids cover the eyes during sleep and protect them from foreign objects or too much light, and spread the tears over their surface.

The nictitating membrane or haw is a transparent sheet that moves sideways across the eye from the inner corner, cleansing and moistening the cornea without shutting out the light. It is found in birds, crocodiles, frogs and fish as well as marsupials like the kangaroo. It is rare in mammals but can be seen in cats and dogs by gently opening the eye when it is asleep. Eyelashes also protect the eyes from the sun and foreign objects.

STRUCTURE OF THE EYE

Lining the eyelids and covering the front of the eyeball is a thin epithelium called the conjunctiva . Conjunctivitis is inflammation of this membrane. Tear glands that open just under the top eyelid secrete a salty solution that keeps the exposed part of the eye moist, washes away dust and contains an enzyme that destroys bacteria.

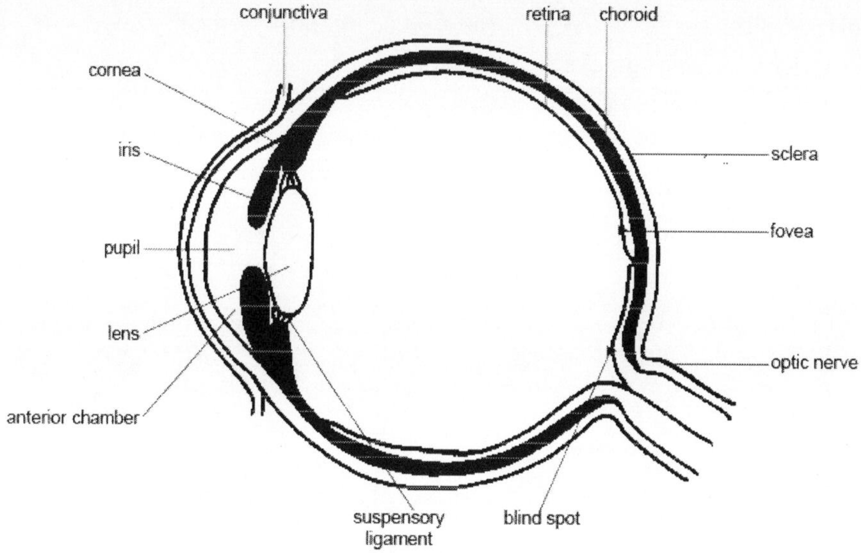

Fig. 14.4

The wall of the eyeball is composed of three layers. From the outside these are the sclera , the choroid and the retina .

The sclera is a tough fibrous layer that protects the eyeball and gives it rigidity. At the front of the eye the sclera is visible as the "white " of the eye, which is modified as the transparent cornea through which the light rays have to pass to enter the eye. The cornea helps focus light that enters the eye.

The choroid lies beneath the sclera. It contains a network of blood vessels that supply the eye with oxygen and nutrients. Its inner surface is highly pigmented and absorbs stray light rays. In nocturnal animals like the cat and possum this highly pigmented layer reflects light as a means of conserving light. This is what makes them shine when caught in car headlights.

At the front of the eye the choroid becomes the iris . This is the coloured part of the eye that controls the amount of light entering the pupil of the eye. In dim light the pupil is wide open so as much light as possible enters while in bright light the pupils contract to protect the retina from damage by excess light.

The pupil in most animals is circular but in many nocturnal animals it is a slit that can close completely. This helps protect the extra-sensitive light sensing tissues of animals like the cat and possum from bright sunlight.

The inner layer lining the inside of the eye is the retina . This contains the light sensing cells called rods and cones.

The rod cells are long and fat and are sensitive to dim light but cannot detect colour. They contain large amounts of a pigment that changes when exposed to light. This pigment comes from vitamin A found in carrots etc. A deficiency of this vitamin causes night blindness. So your mother was right when she told you to eat your carrots as they would help you see in the dark!

The cone cells provide colour vision and allow animals to see details. Most are found in the centre of the retina and they are most densely concentrated in a small area called the fovea . This is the area of sharpest vision, where the words you are reading at this moment are focussed on your retina.

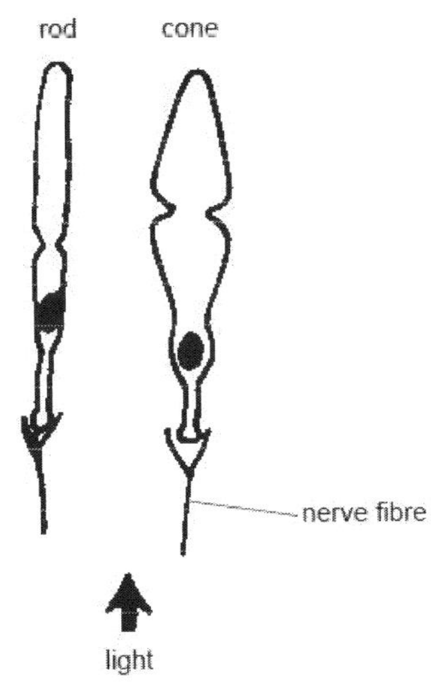

Fig. 14.5

Diagram 15.5 - A rod and cone from the retina

The nerve fibres from the cells of the retina join and leave the eye via the optic nerve . There are no rods or cones here and it is a blind spot . The optic nerve passes through the back of the orbit and enters the brain.

The lens is situated just behind the pupil and the iris. It is a crystalline structure with no blood vessels and is held in position by a ligament. This is attached to a muscle, which changes the shape of the lens so both near and distant objects can be focussed by the eye. This ability to change the focus of the lens is called accommodation . In many mammals the muscles that bring about accommodation are poorly developed, Rats, cows and dogs, for example, are thought to be unable to focus clearly on near objects.

In old age and certain diseases the lens may become cloudy resulting in blurred vision. This is called a cataract . Within the eyeball are two cavities, the anterior and posterior chambers , separated by the lens. They contain fluids the aqueous and vitreous hu- mours respectively, that maintain the shape of the eyeball and help press the retina firmly against the choroid so clear images are seen.

How The Eye Sees

Eyes work quite like a camera. Light rays from an object enter the eye and are focused on the retina (the "film") at the back of the eye. The cornea, the lens and the fluid within the eye all help to focus the light. They do this by bending the light rays so that light from the object falls on the retina. This bending of light is called refraction . The light stimulates the light sensitive cells of the retina and nerve impulses are produced that pass down the optic nerve to the brain.

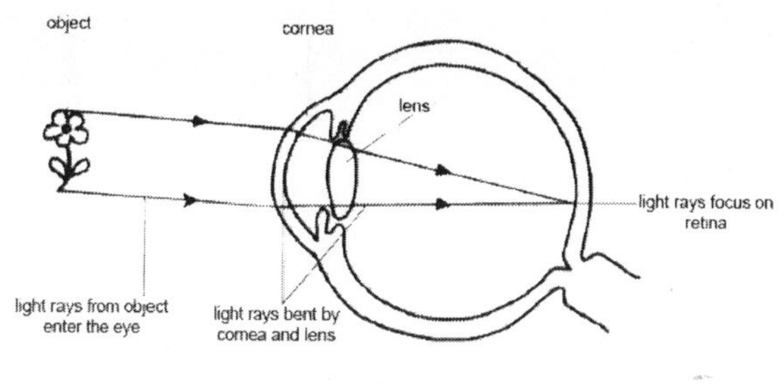

Fig. 14.6

Colour Vision In Animals

As mentioned before, the retina has two different kinds of cells that are stimulated by light- rods and cones. In humans and higher primates like baboons and gorillas the rods function in dim light and do not perceive colour, while the cones are stimulated by bright light and perceive details and colour.

Other mammals have very few cones in their retinas and it is believed that they see no or only a limited range of colour. It is, of course, difficult to find out exactly what animals do see. It is thought that deer, rats, and rabbits and nocturnal animals like the cat are colour-blind, and dogs probably see green and blue. Some fish and most birds seem to have better colour vision than humans and they use colour, often very vivid ones, for recognizing each other as well as for courtship and protection.

Binocular Vision

Animals like cats that hunt have eyes placed on the front of the head in such a way that both eyes see the same wide area but from slightly different angles. This is called binocular vision. Its main advantage is that it enables the animals to estimate the distance to the prey so they can chase it and pounce accurately.

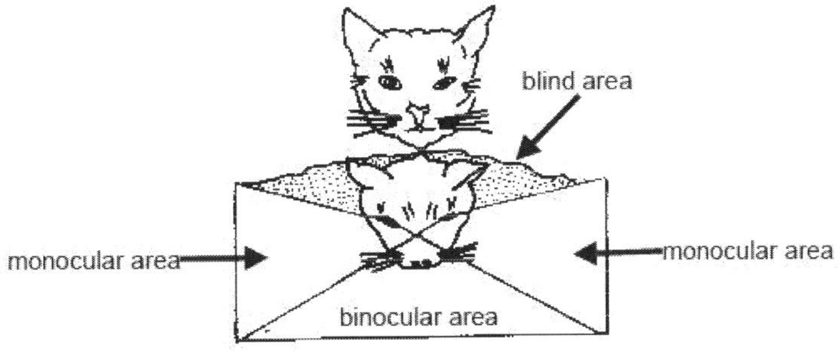

Fig. 14.7

In contrast plant-eating prey animals like the rabbit and deer need to have a wide panoramic view so they can see predators approaching. They therefore have eyes placed on the side of the head, each with its own field of vision. They have only a very small area of binocular vision in front of the head but are extremely sensitive to movement.

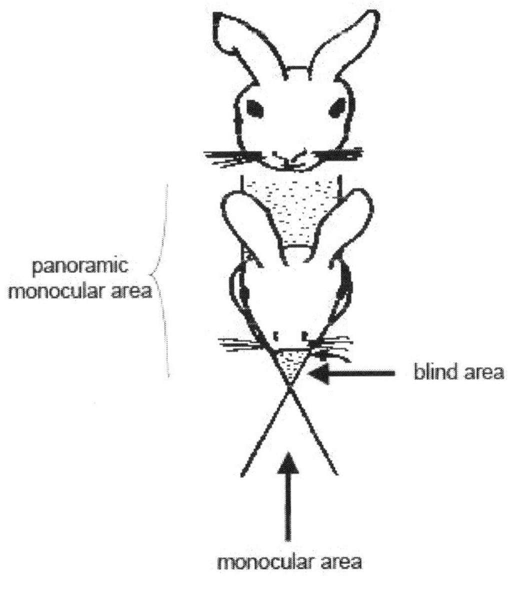

Fig. 14.8

HEARING

Animals use the sense of hearing for many different purposes. It is used to sense danger and enemies, to detect prey, to identify prospective mates and to communicate within social groups. Some animals (e.g. most bats and dolphins) use sound to "see" by echolocation. By sending out a cry and interpreting the echo, they sense obstacles or potential prey.

Structure of the Ear

Most of the ear, the organ of hearing, is hidden from view within the boney skull. It consists of three main regions: the outer ear, the middle ear and the inner ear.

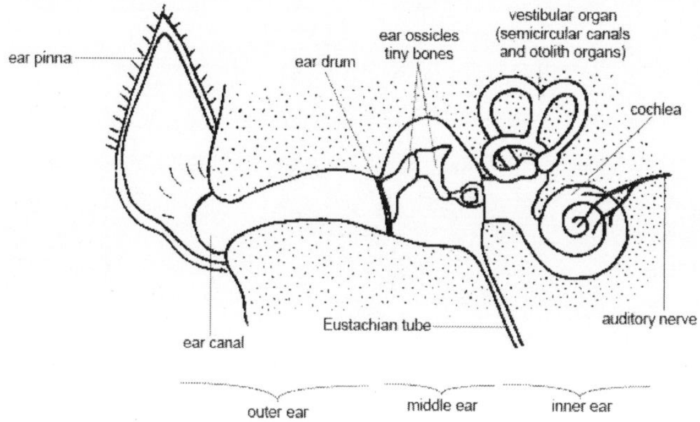

Fig. 14.9

The outer ear consists of an ear canal leading inwards to a thin membrane known as the eardrum or tympanic membrane that stretches across the canal. Many animals have an external ear flap or pinna to collect and funnel the sound into the ear canal. The pinnae (plural of pinna) usually face forwards on the head but many animals can swivel them towards the source of the sound.

In dogs the ear canal is long and bent and often traps wax or provides an ideal habitat for mites, yeast and bacteria.

The middle ear consists of a cavity in the skull that is connected to the pharynx (throat) by a long narrow tube called the Eustachian tube . This links the middle ear to the outside air so that the air pressure on both sides of the eardrum can be kept the same. Everyone knows the uncomfortable feeling (and affected hearing) that occurs when you drive down a steep hill and the unequal air pressures on the two sides of the eardrum cause it to distort. The discomfort is relieved when you swallow because the Eustachian tubes open and the pressure on either side equalises.

Within the cavity of the middle ear are three of the smallest bones in the body, the auditory ossicles. They are known as the hammer, the anvil and the stirrup because of their resemblance to the shape of these objects. These tiny bones articulate (move against) each other and transfer the vibrations of the eardrum to the membrane covering the opening to the inner ear.

The inner ear is a complicated series of fluid-filled tubes imbedded in the bone of the skull. It consists of two main parts. These are the cochlea where sound waves are converted to nerve impulses and the vestibular organ that is associated with the sense of balance and has no role in hearing (see later).

The cochlea looks rather like a coiled up snail shell. Within it there are specialised cells with fine hairs on their surface that respond to the movement of the fluid within the cochlea by producing nervous impulses that travel to the brain along the auditory nerve .

HOW THE EAR HEARS

Sound waves can be thought of as vibrations in the air. They are collected by the ear pinna and pass down the ear canal where they cause the eardrum to vibrate. (An interesting fact is that when you are listening to someone speaking your eardrum vibrates at exactly the same rate as the vocal cords of the person speaking to you).

The vibration of the eardrum sets the three tiny bones in the middle ear moving against each other so that the vibration is transferred to the membrane covering the opening to the inner ear. As well as transferring the vibration, the tiny ear bones also amplify it. The three tiny bones are called the stirrup, anvil, and hammer. They were called such of their form. In the human ear this amplification is about 20 times while in desert-dwelling animals like the kangaroo rat it is 100 times. This acute hearing warns them of the approach of predators like owls and snakes, even in the dark.

- The vibration causes waves in the fluid in the inner ear that pass down the cochlea. These waves stimulate the tiny hair cells to produce nerve impulses that travel via the auditory nerve to the cerebral cortex of the brain where they are interpreted as sound.
- To summarise: The route sound waves take as they pass through the ear is: External ear | tympanic membrane | ear ossicles | inner ear |cochlear | hair cells
- The hair cells generate a nerve impulse that travels down the auditory nerve to the brain.
- Remember that sound waves do not pass along the Eustachian tube. Its function is to equalise the air pressure on either side of the tympanic membrane.

Balance

The vestibular organ of the inner ear helps an animal maintain its posture and keep balanced by monitoring the movement and position of the head. It consists of two structures- the semicircular canals and the otolith organs .

The semicircular canals respond to movement of the body. They tell an animal whether it is moving up or down, left or right. They consist of three canals set in three different planes at right angles to each other so that movement in any direction can be registered. The canals contain fluid and sense cells with fine hairs that project into the fluid. When the head moves the fluid swirls in the canals and stimulates the hair cells. These send nerve impulses along the vestibular nerve to the cerebellum .

Note that the semicircular canals register acceleration and deceleration as well as changes in direction but do not respond to movement that is at a constant speed.

The otolith organs are sometimes known as gravity receptors. They tell you if your head is tilted or if you are standing on your head. They consist of bulges at the base of the semi circular canals that contain hair cells that are covered by a mass of jelly containing tiny pieces of chalk called otoliths (see diagram 15.10). When the head is tilted, or moved suddenly, the otoliths pull on the hair cells, which produce a nerve impulse. This travels down the vestibular nerve to the cerebellum . By coordinating the nerve impulses from the semicircular canals and otolith organs the cerebellum helps the animal keep its balance.

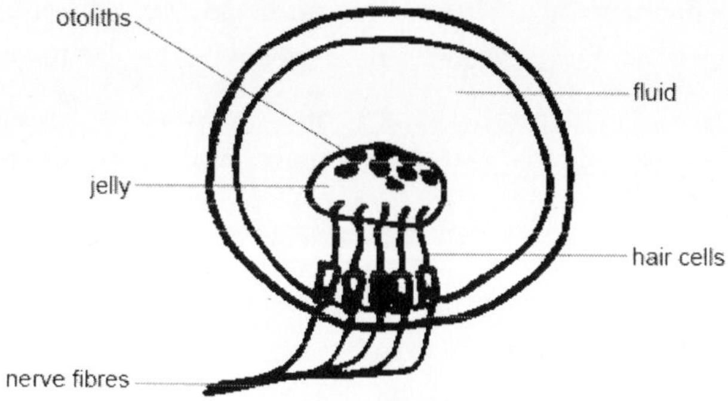

Figure 14.10

Test Yourself

1. Where are the organs that sense pain, pressure and temperature found?
2. Which sense organ responds to chemicals in the air?
3. Match the words in the list below with the following descriptions.

optic nerve | choroid | cornea | aqueous humor | retina | cones | iris | vitreous humour | sclera | lens

a) Focuses light rays on the retina.
b) Respond to colour and detail.
c) Outer coat of the eyeball.
d) Carries nerve impulses from the retina to the brain.
e) The chamber behind the lens is filled with this.
f) This layer of the eyeball reflects light in nocturnal animals like the cat.
g) This is the transparent window at the front of the eye.
h) This constricts in bright light to reduce the amount of light entering the eye.
i) The light rays are focused on here by the lens and cornea.
j) The chamber in front of the lens is filled with this.

15

ENDOCRINE SYSTEM

In order to survive, animals must constantly adapt to changes in the environment. The nervous and endocrine systems both work together to bring about this adaptation. In general the nervous system responds rapidly to short-term changes by sending electrical impulses along nerves and the endocrine system brings about longer-term adaptations by sending out chemical messengers called hormones into the blood stream.

For example, think about what happens when a male and female cat meet under your bedroom window at night. The initial response of both cats may include spitting, fighting and spine tingling yowling - all brought about by the nervous system. Fear and stress then activates the adrenal glands to secrete the hormone adrenaline which increases the heart and respiratory rates. If mating occurs, other hormones stimulate the release of ova from the ovary of the female and a range of different hormones maintains pregnancy, delivery of the kittens and lactation.

ENDOCRINE GLANDS AND HORMONES

Hormones are chemicals that are secreted by endocrine glands . Unlike exocrine glands, endocrine glands have no ducts, but release their secretions directly into the blood system, which carries them throughout the body. However, hormones only affect the specific target organs that recognize them. For example, although it is carried to virtually every cell in the body, follicle stimulating hormone (FSH), released from the anterior pituitary gland , only acts on the follicle cells of the ovaries causing them to develop.

A nerve impulse travels rapidly and produces an almost instantaneous response but one that lasts only briefly. In contrast, hormones act more slowly and their effects may be long lasting. Target cells respond to minute quantities of hormones and the concentration in the blood is always extremely low. However, target cells are sensitive to subtle changes in hormone concentration and the endocrine system regulates processes by changing the rate of hormone secretion.

The main endocrine glands in the body are the pituitary, pineal, thyroid, parathyroid and adrenal glands , the pancreas, ovaries and testes.

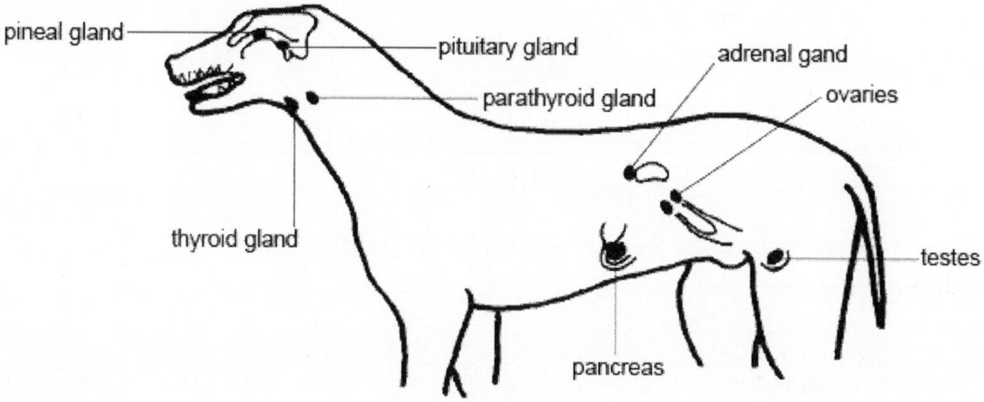

Fig.15.1

The Pituitary Gland And Hypothalamus

The pituitary gland is a pea-sized structure that is attached by a stalk to the underside of the cerebrum of the brain. It is often called the "master" endocrine gland because it controls many of the other endocrine glands in the body. However, we now know that the pituitary gland is itself controlled by the hypothalamus . This small but vital region of the brain lies just above the pituitary and provides the link between the nervous and endocrine systems. It controls the autonomic nervous system , produces a range of hormones and regulates the secretion of many others from the pituitary gland.

The pituitary gland is divided into two parts with different functions - the anterior and posterior pituitary.

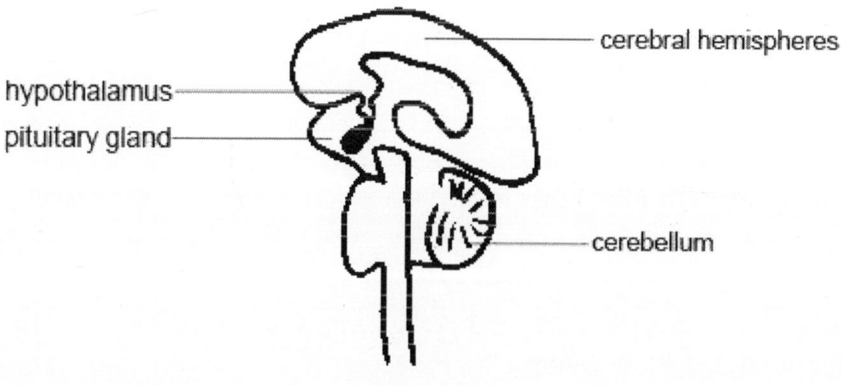

Fig. 15.2

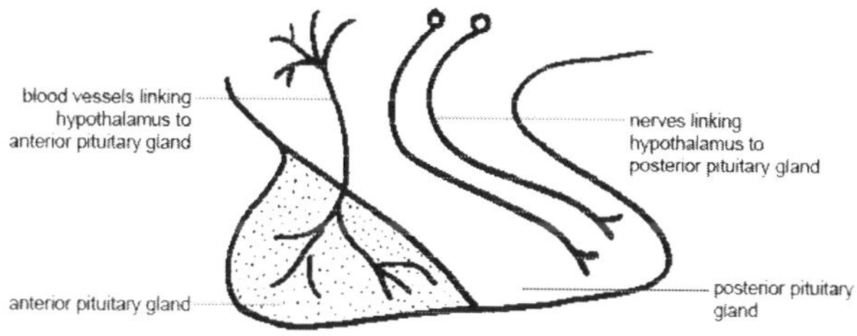

Fig.15.3

The anterior pituitary gland secretes hormones that regulate a wide range of activities in the body. These include:

1. Growth hormone that stimulates body growth.
2. Prolactin that initiates milk production.
3. Follicle stimulating hormone (FSH) that stimulates the development of the follicles of the ovaries. These then secrete oestrogen.
4. melanocyte stimulating hormone (MSH) that causes darkening of skin by producing melanin
5. lutenizing hormone (LH) that stimulates ovulation and production of progesterone and testosterone

THE PINEAL GLAND

The pineal gland is found deep within the brain. It is sometimes known as the 'third eye" as it responds to light and day length. It produces the hormone melatonin which influences the development of sexual maturity and the seasonality of breeding and hibernation bright light inhibits melatonin secretion low level of melatonin in bright light makes one feel good and these increases fertility High level of melatonin in deam light makes an animal tired and depressed therefore low fertility in animals

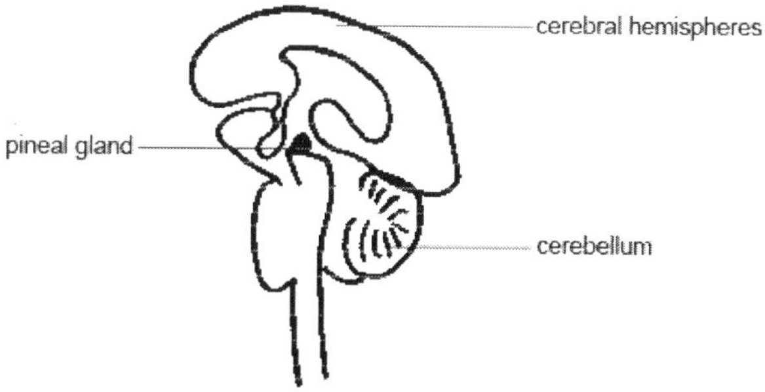

Fig. 15.4

The Thyroid Gland

The thyroid gland is situated in the neck, just in front of the windpipe or trachea. It produces the hormone thyroxine , which influences the rate of growth and development of young animals. In mature animals it increases the rate of chemical reactions in the body.

Thyroxine consists of 60% iodine and too little in the diet can cause goitre , an enlargement of the thyroid gland. Many inland soils in New Zealand contain almost no iodine so goitre can be common in stock when iodine supplements are not given. To add to the problem, chemicals called goitrogens that occur naturally in plants like kale that belong to the cabbage family , can also cause goitre even when there is adequate iodine available.

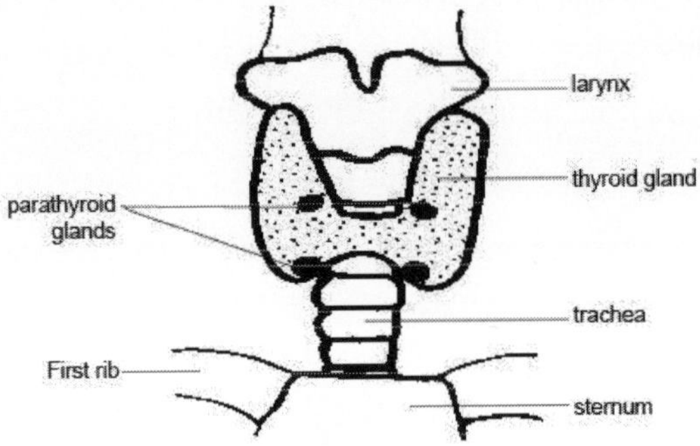

Fig. 15.5

THE PARATHYROID GLANDS

The parathyroid glands are also found in the neck just behind the thyroid glands. They produce the hormone parathormone that regulates the amount of calcium in the blood and influences the excretion of phosphates in the urine.

The Adrenal Gland

The adrenal glands are situated on the cranial surface of the kidneys. There are two parts to this endocrine gland, an outer cortex and an inner medulla .

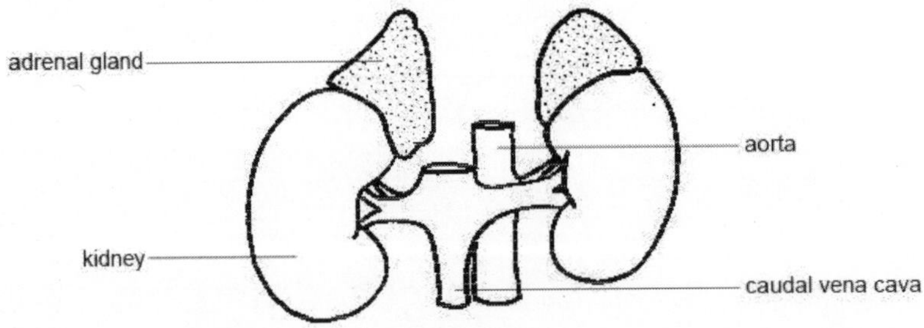

Fig.15.6

The adrenal cortex produces several hormones. These include:

1. Aldosterone that regulates the concentration of sodium and potassium in the blood by controlling the amounts that are secreted or reabsorbed in the kidney tubules.

2. Cortisone and hydrocortisone (cortisol) that have complex effects on glucose, protein and fat metabolism. In general they increase metabolism. They are also often administered to animals to counteract allergies and for treating arthritic and rheumatic conditions. However, prolonged use should be avoided if possible as they can increase weight and reduce the ability to heal.
3. Male and female sex hormones similar to those secreted by the ovaries and testes.

The hormones secreted by the adrenal cortex also play a part in "general adaptation syndrome " which occurs in situations of prolonged stress.

The adrenal medulla secretes adrenalin (also called epinephrine). Adrenalin is respon- sible for the so-called flight fight, fright response that prepares the animal for emergencies. Faced with a perilous situation the animal needs to either fight or make a rapid escape. To do either requires instant energy, particularly in the skeletal muscles. Adrenaline increases the amount of blood reaching them by causing their blood vessels to dilate and the heart to beat faster. An increased rate of breathing increases the amount of oxygen in the blood and glucose is released from the liver to provide the fuel for energy production. Sweating increases to keep the muscles cool and the pupils of the eye dilate so the animal has a wide field of view. Functions like digestion and urine production that are not critical to immediate survival slow down as blood vessels to these parts constrict.

Note that the effects of adrenalin are similar to those of the sympathetic nervous system.

The Pancreas

In most animals the pancreas is an oblong, pinkish organ that lies in the first bend of the small intestine. In rodents and rabbits, however, it is spread thinly through the mesentery and is sometimes difficult to see.

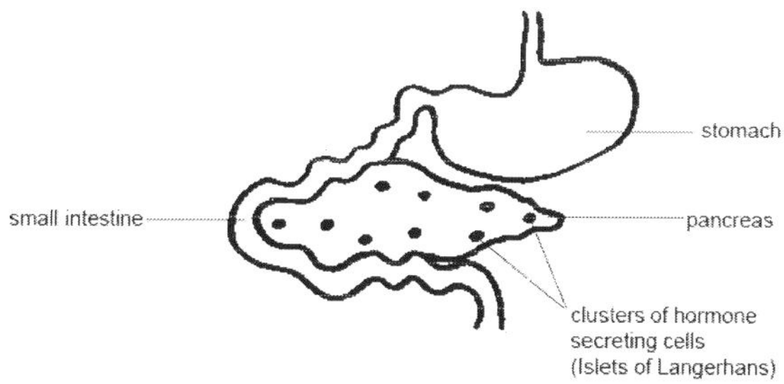

Fig. 15.7

Most of the pancreas acts as an exocrine gland producing digestive enzymes that are secreted into the small intestine. The endocrine part of the organ consists of small clusters of cells (called Islets of Langerhans) that secrete the hormone insulin . This hormone regulates the amount of glucose in the blood by increasing the rate at which glucose is converted to glycogen in the liver and the movement of glucose from the blood into cells.

In diabetes mellitus the pancreas produces insufficient insulin and glucose levels in the blood can increase to a dangerous level. A major symptom of this condition is glucose in the urine.

THE OVARIES

The ovaries, located in the lower abdomen, produce two important sex hormones.

1. The follicle cells , under the influence of FSH (see the pituitary gland above), pro- duce oestrogen , which stimulates the development of female sexual characteristics - the mammary glands, generally smaller build of female animals etc. It also stimulates the thickening of the lining of the uterus in preparation for pregnancy.
2. Progesterone is produced by the corpus luteum, the endocrine gland that develops in the empty follicle following ovulation. It promotes the further preparation of the uterine lining for pregnancy and prevents the uterus contracting until the baby is born.

The Testes

Cells around the sperm producing ducts of the testis produce the hormone testosterone. This stimulates the development of the male reproductive system and the male sexual characteristics - generally larger body of male animals, mane in lions, tusks in boars, etc

Homeostasis and Feedback Control

Animals can only survive if the environment within their bodies and their cells is kept constant and independent of the changing conditions in the external environment. As mentioned in module 1.6, the process by which this stability is maintained is called homeostasis. The body achieves this stability by constantly monitoring the internal conditions and if they deviate from the norm initiating processes that bring them back to it. This mechanism is called feedback control. For example, to maintain a constant body temperature the hypothalamus monitors the blood temperature and initiates processes that increase or decrease heat production by the body and loss from the skin so the optimum temperature is always maintained. The processes involved in the control of body temperature, water balance, blood loss and acid/base balance are summarized below.

1. Temperature control

The biochemical and physiological processes in the cell are sensitive to temperature. The optimum body temperature is about 37C [99F] for mammals, and about 40C [104F] for birds. Biochemical processes in the cells, particularly in muscles and the liver, produce heat. The heat is distributed through the body by the blood and is lost mainly through the skin surface. The production of this heat and its loss through the skin is controlled by the hypothalamus in the brain which acts rather like a thermostat on an electric heater. .

(a) When the body temperature rises above the optimum, a decrease in temperature is achieved by:

- Sweating and panting to increase heat loss by evaporation.
- Expansion of the blood vessels near the skin surface so heat is lost to the air.
- Reducing muscle exertion to the minimum.

(b) When the body temperature falls below the optimum, an increase in temperature can be achieved by:

- Moving to a heat source e.g. in the sun, out of the wind.
- Increasing muscular activity

Summary of Homeostatic Mechanisms

- Shivering
- Making the hair stand on end by contraction of the hair erector muscles or fluffing of the feathers so there is an insulating layer of air around the body
- Constricting the blood vessels near the skin surface so heat loss to the air is decreased

2. Water balance

The concentration of the body fluids remains relatively constant irrespective of the diet or the quantity of water taken into the body by the animal. Water is lost from the body by many routes but the kidney is the main organ that influences the quantity that is lost. Again it is the hypothalamus that monitors the concentration of the blood and initiates the release of hormones from the posterior pituitary gland. These act on the kidney tubules to influence the amount of water (and sodium ions) absorbed from the fluid flowing along them.

(a) When the body fluids become too concentrated and the osmotic pressure too high, water retention in the kidney tubules can be achieved by:

- An increased production of antidiuretic hormone (ADH) from the posterior pituitary gland, which causes more water to be reabsorbed from the kidney tubules.
- A decreased blood pressure in the glomerulus of the kidney results in less fluid filtering through into the kidney tubules so less urine is produced.

(b) When the body fluids become too dilute and the osmotic pressure too low, water loss in the urine can be achieved by:

- A decrease in the secretion of ADH, so less water is reabsorbed from the kidney tubules and more diluted urine is produced.
- An increase in the blood pressure in the glomerulus so more fluid filters into the kidney tubule and more urine is produced.
- An increase in sweating or panting that also increases the amount of water lost.

Another hormone, aldosterone, secreted by the cortex of the adrenal gland, also affects water balance indirectly. It does this by increasing the absorption of sodium ions (Na-) from the kidney tubules. This increases water retention since it increases the osmotic pressure of the fluids around the tubules and water therefore flows out of them by osmosis.

3. Maintenance of blood volume after moderate blood loss

Loss of blood or body fluids leads to decreased blood volume and hence decreased blood pressure. The result is that the blood system fails to deliver enough oxygen and nutrients to the cells, which stop functioning properly and may die. Cells of the brain are particularly vulnerable. This condition is known as shock.

If blood loss is not extreme, various mechanisms come into play to compensate and ensure permanent tissue damage does not occur. These mechanisms include:

- Increased thirst and drinking increases blood volume.
- Blood vessels in the skin and kidneys constrict to reduce the total volume of the blood system and hence retain blood pressure.
- Heart rate increases. This also increases blood pressure.
- Antidiuretic hormone (ADH) is released by the posterior pituitary gland. This increases water re-absorption in the collecting ducts of the kidney tubules so concentrated urine is produced and water loss is reduced. This helps maintain blood volume.
- Loss of fluid causes an increase in osmotic pressure of the blood. Proteins, mainly albumin, released into the blood by the liver further increase the osmotic pressure causing fluid from the tissues to be drawn into the blood by osmosis. This increases blood volume.
- Aldosterone, secreted by the adrenal cortex, increases the absorption of sodium ions (Na-) and water from the kidney tubules. This increases urine concentration and helps retain blood volume.

If blood or fluid loss is extreme and the blood volume falls by more than 15-25%, the above mechanisms are unable to compensate and the condition of the animal progressively deteriorates. The animal will die unless a vet administers fluid or blood.

4. Acid/ base balance

Biochemical reactions within the body are very sensitive to even small changes in acidity or alkalinity (i.e. pH) and any departure from the narrow limits disrupts the functioning of the cells. It is therefore important that the blood contains balanced quantities of acids and bases.

The normal pH of blood is in the range 7.35 to 7.45 and there are a number of mechanisms that operate to maintain the pH in this range. Breathing is one of these mechanisms.

Much of the carbon dioxide produced by respiration in cells is carried in the blood as carbonic acid. As the amount of carbon dioxide in the blood increases the blood becomes more acidic and the pH decreases. This is called acidosis and when severe can cause coma and death. On the other hand, alkalosis (blood that is too alkaline) causes over stimulation of the nervous system and when severe can lead to convulsions and death.

(a) When vigorous activity generating large quantities of carbon dioxide causes the blood to becomes too acidic it can be counteracted in two ways:

- By the rapid removal of carbon dioxide from the blood by deep, panting breaths
  By the secretion of hydrogen ions (H+) into the urine by the kidney tubules.

(b) When over breathing or hyperventilation results in low levels of carbon dioxide in the blood and the blood is too alkaline, various mechanisms come into play to bring the pH back to within the normal range. These include:

- A slower rate of breathing
- A reduction in the amount of hydrogen ions (H+) secreted into the urine.

16

REPRODUCTIVE SYSTEM

The reproductive system is a collection of internal and external organs — in both males and females — that work together for the purpose of procreating, according to the Cleveland Clinic. Due to its vital role in the survival of the species, many scientists argue that the reproductive system is among the most important systems in the entire body.

Animal reproduction specialists can play a vital role in the survival of endangered animal species, as well as developing programs for production or performance animals, or working with breeders. Your role could involve artificial insemination and other assisted breeding technologies, or you may be more concerned with monitoring, measuring and assessing breeding patterns in animal populations.

As an animal reproduction specialist, you could:

- Develop breeding plans for endangered species
- Manage captive animal populations
- Work with livestock animals and horses on farms and studs.

Depending on your interests, you could work with animals from domestic breeds competing at shows, to performance animals, livestock, or animals in zoos and wildlife parks in Australia and internationally. Your career could improve genetic diversity in a production or captive animal population, or help bring a species back from the brink of extinction.

Animal reproduction experts could also study animal behaviour, examining how animals choose mates, care for offspring or avoid predators. As a specialist in this area, your workplace could be a zoo, research laboratory, animal shelter or veterinary hospital.

THE MALE REPRODUCTIVE SYSTEM

One of the fundamental laws of nature is that every species makes a vigorous attempt to reproduce its kind. The higher animals reproduce sexually. This involves the production of potentially differentiated sex cells by the male and female. In animals, this has led to the development of highly specialized body parts for the specific purpose of reproduction.

The primary sex organs of the male are the two testes, which are normally located in an external sac of skin called the scrotum. The secondary sex organs are the duct system (the vas deferens), the epididymis, and the penis. The penis is trans-versed by the urethra, which is common passageway for urine and semen. The semen is composed of sexual secretions and spermatozoa. Besides the reproductive tract, there are a few accessory organs like the prostate gland, a pair of seminal vesicles, and two Cowper's glands, or bulbo-urethral glands. The primary, secondary and accessory sex organs are collectively called male reproductive tract.

The male reproductive system consists of a pair of testes that produce sperm (or spermatozoa), ducts that transport the sperm to the penis and glands that add secretions to the sperm to make semen.

The various parts of the male reproductive system with a summary of their functions are shown in Fig. 16.1.

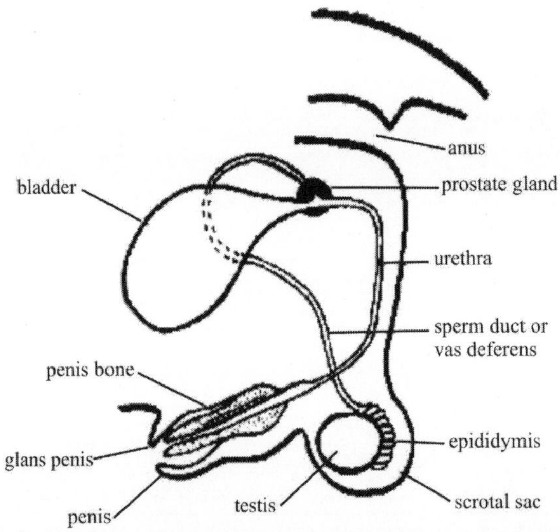

Fig. 16.1 The Reproductive Organs of a Male Dog.

Semen consists of 10% sperm and 90% fluid and as sperm pass down the ducts from testis to penis, (accessory) glands add various secretion. . .

Accessory Glands

Three different glands may be involved in producing the secretions in which sperm are suspended, although the number and type of glands varies from species to species.

Seminal vesicles are important in rats, bulls, boars and stallions but are absent in cats and dogs. When present they produce secretions that make up much of the volume of the semen, and transport and provide nutrients for the sperm.

The prostate gland is important in dogs and humans. It produces an alkaline secretion that neutralizes the acidity of the male urethra and female vagina.

Cowper's glands (bulbourethral glands) have various functions in different species. The secretions may lubricate, flush out urine or form a gelatinous plug that traps the semen in the female reproductive system after copulation and prevents other males of the same species fertilizing an already mated female. Cowper's glands are absent in bears and aquatic mammals.

Testes

The testes are the primary organs of reproduction in males, just as ovaries are primary organs of reproduction in females. Testes are considered primary because they produce male gametes (spermatozoa) and male sex hormones (androgens). Testes differ from ovaries in that al potential gametes are not present at birth. Germ cells, located in the seminiferous tubules, undergo continual cell divisions, forming new spermatozoa throughout the normal reproductive life of the male.

Testes also differ from ovaries in that they do not remain in the body cavity. They decend from their site of origin, near the kidneys, down through the inguinal into the scrotum. Descent of the testes occurs because of an apparent shortening of the gubernaculum, a ligament extending from the inguinal region and attaching to the tail the epididymis. This apparent shortening occurs because the gubernaculum does not grow as rapidly as the body wall. The testes are drawn closer to the inguinal cannals and intra-abdominal pressure adis passage of the testes through the inguinal cannals into the scrotum. Both gonadotropic of hormones and androgens regulate descent of the testes. This descent is completed in the fetus by midpregnancy in cattle and just before birth in horses. In some cases one or both testes fail to descend due to a defect in development. If neither descends, the animal is termed a biaterral crytorchid. Bilateral cryptochids are sterile. if only one testis descends he is a unilateral cryptochid. The unilateral cyptochid is usually fertile due to the descended testis. The cyptochid condition can be corrected by surgery, but this is not recommended for farm animals. The condition can be inherited;therefore, surgical correction would result in the perpetuation of an undesirable trait.

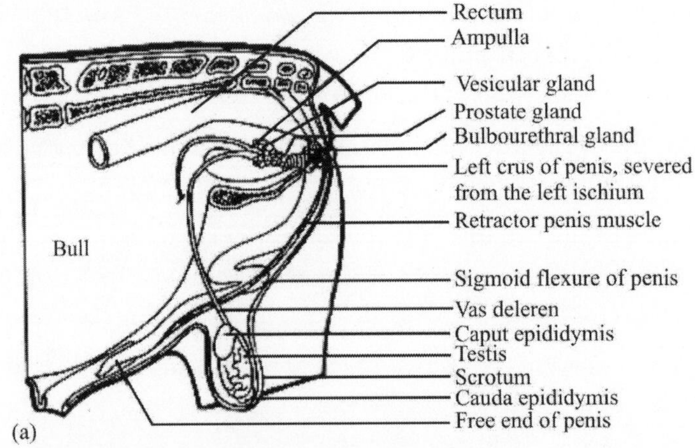

Fig. 16.2 a

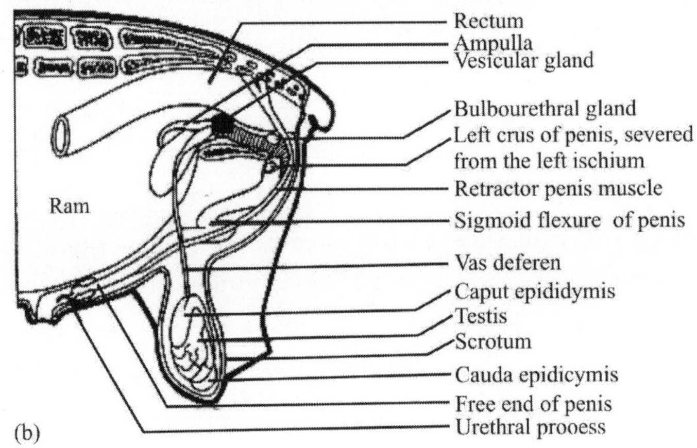

Fig. 16.2 b

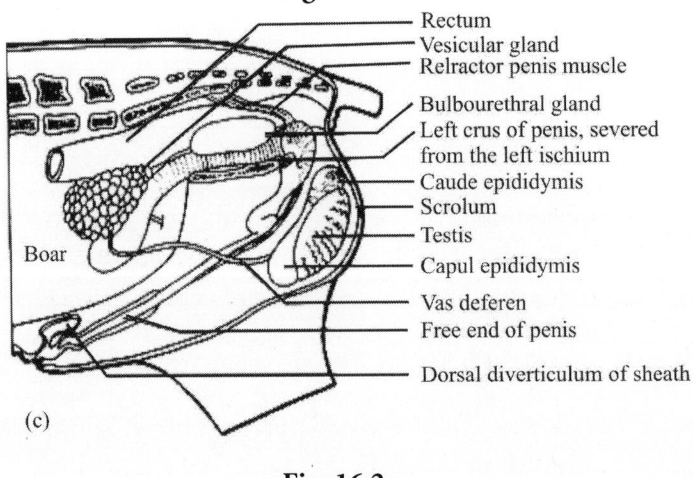

Fig. 16.2 c

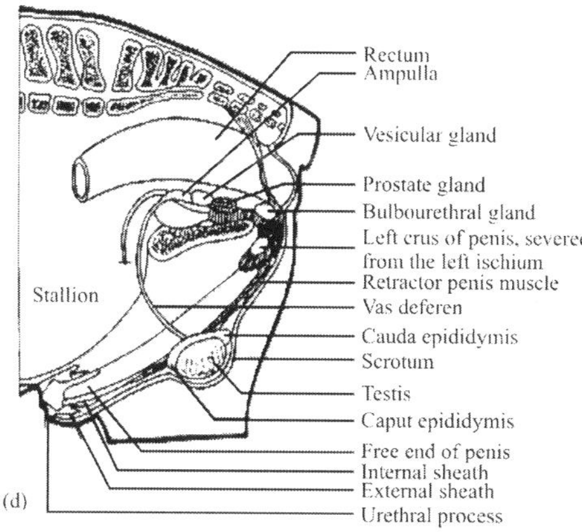

Fig. 16.2 Diagram of the Reproductive System of The (a) Bull; (b) Ram; (c) Boar; and (d) Stallion.

Sperm need temperatures between 2 to 10 degrees Centigrade lower and then the body temperature to develop. This is the reason why the testes are located in a bag of skin called the scrotal sacs (or scrotum) that hangs below the body and where the evaporation of secretions from special glands can further reduce the temperature. In many animals (including humans) the testes descend into the scrotal sacs at birth but in some animals they do not descend until sexual maturity and in others they only descend temporarily during the breeding season. A mature animal in which one or both testes have not descended is called a cryptorchid and is usually infertile.

The problem of keeping sperm at a low enough temperature is even greater in birds that have a higher body temperature than mammals. For this reason bird's sperm are usually produced at night when the body temperature is lower and the sperm themselves are more resistant to heat.

The testes consist of a mass of coiled tubes (the seminiferous or sperm producing tubules) in which the sperm are formed by meiosis. Cells lying between the seminiferous tubules produce the male sex hormone testosterone.

When the sperm are mature they accumulate in the collecting ducts and then pass to the epididymisbefore moving to the sperm duct or vas deferens. The two sperm ducts join the urethra just below the bladder, which passes through the penis and transports both sperm and urine.

Ejaculation discharges the semen from the erect penis. It is brought about by the contraction of the epididymis, vas deferens, prostate gland and urethra.

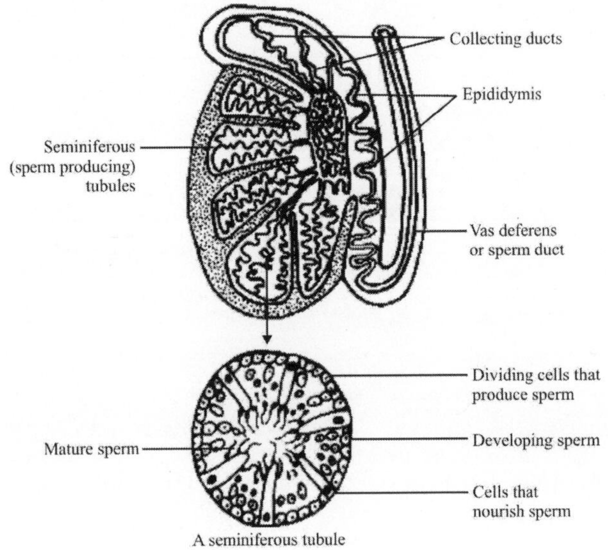

Fig. 16.3 The Testis and a Magnified Seminiferous Tubule.

Functional Morphology

The testis of the bull is 10 to 13 cm long, 5 to 6. 5 cm wide and weighs 300 to 400 gm. THe testis is of similar size in boars, but is smaller in rams, bucks (goats), and stallions.

In all species testes are covered with the tunica vaginalis, a serous tissue, which is an extension of the peritoneum. This serous coat is obtained as the testes descend into the scrotum and is attached along the line of the epididymis. The outer layer of the testes, the tunica albuginea testis, is a thin white memberane of elastic connective tissue. Numberous blood vesselsare visible just nuder its surface. Beneath the tunica albuginea testis is the parenchyma, the functional layer of the testes. The parenchyma has a yellowish color and is divided into segments by incomplete septa of connective tissue. Located within these segments of parenchyma tissue are the seminiferous tubules. Seminiferous tubules are formed from primary sex cords. They contains germcells(spermatogonia) and nursa cells (Sertolicells). Sertoli cells are larger and less numberous thanspermatogonia. With stimulation by FSH, Sertoli cells produce both androgen binding protein and inhibin. Seminiferous tubules are the site of spermatozoa production. They are small, convoluted tubules approxilately 200m in diameter. It has been estimated that the seminiferous tubules from a pair of bull testes, streched out and laid end, approach 5 km in length. They make up 80% of the weight of the testes. seminiferous tubules join a network of tubules, the rete testis, which connects to 12 to 15 small ducts, the vasa efferential. which converge into the head of the epididymis.

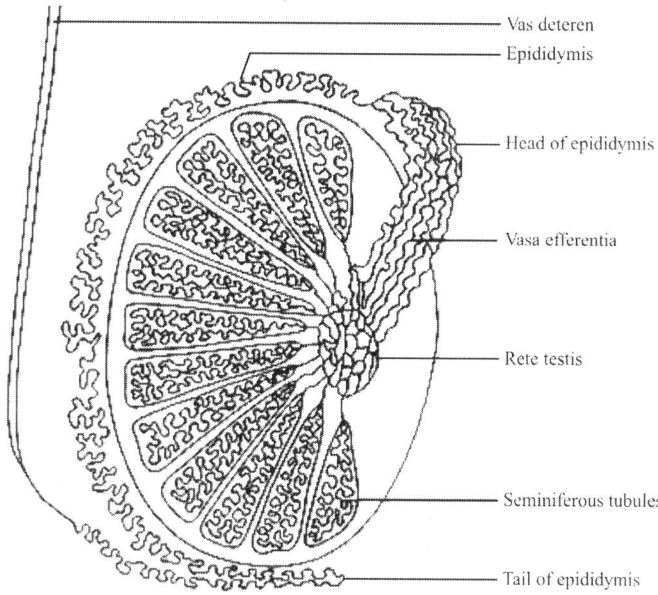

Fig. 16.4 Sagittal Section of Testis Illustratingsegments of Parenchymal Tissue which Contain the Seminiferous Tubules, Rete testis, vasa Efferentis, Epididymis, and Scrotal Portion of the Vas Deferen.

Leydig (interstitial) cells are found in the parenchyma of the testes between the seminiferous tubules. LH timulates Leydig cells to produce testosterone and small quantities of dther androgens.

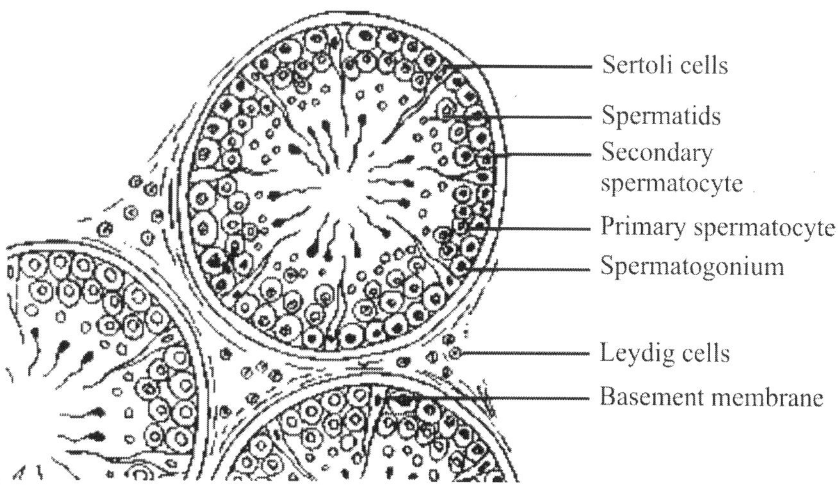

Fig. 16.5 Cross Section of Parenchymal Tissue Showing Relationship between the Seminiferous Tubules and Interstitial Tissue Containing Leydig Cells.

Testosterone is needed for development of secondary sex characteristics and for normal mating behavior. In addition, it is necessary for the function of the accessary glands, production of spermatozoa and maintenance of the male duct system. Through its effects on the male, testosterone aids in maintenance of optimumcondtions for spermatogenesis, transprot of spermatozoa and deposition of spermatozoa into the female tract. Normal body temperature will not affect the function of the Leydig cells. For example, bilaterial crytochids develop secondary sex characteristics, have normal sexual vigor, and can do all things associated with reproduction exceptrpoduction of spromatozoa.

SCROTUM AND SPERMATIC CORD

The scrotum is two-lobed sac which enclosed the testes. It is located in the inguinal region between the rear legs of most species. The scrotum has the same embryonic origin as the labia majora in the female. It is composed of an outer layer of think skin with numerous large sweat and sebaceous glands. This outer is lined is with a layer of smooth muscle fibers, the tunica dartos, which is interspersed with connective tissue. The tunica dartos divides the scrotum into two pouches, and is attached to the tunica vagimals at the bottom of each pouch.

The spermatic cordconeects the testis to its life support mechanisms, the convoluted testicular arteries and surrounding venus plexus, and nerve trunks. In addition, the spermatic cord is composed of smooth muscle fibers, connective tissue, and a portion of the vas deferens. Both the spermatic cords and scrotum contribute to the support of the testes. Also, they have a joint function in regulating the temperature of the testes.

Temperature Control

Serveral examples can be given to illustrate the inportance of temperature control of the testes. If a ram, s scrotum is insulated, or the testes are tied against the abdomen, sterility results. The higher temperature causes degeneration of the cells lining the wall of the seminiferous tubules. Fetility will be restored if the testes and scrotum are returned to their natural state before total degeneration occurs. However, a few weeks will be required before fertile semen is again produced. (Sometimes men with high fevers are sterile for short period after recovery.) The bilateral crytorchid is sterile, again illustrating that production of spermatozoa stops when the temperature inside the testes is as high normal body temperature.

Low fertility semen produced by several species of farm animals during the summer has been attributes to the inability of the body, s cooing mechanisms to keep the testes cool enough. In cattle, when ambient temperaturesrange from 5°C to 21°C, the temperature inside the testes will be about 4°C below body temperature (38. 6°C). As the ambient temperature increasea to approximately 38°C, the temperature of both body and the testes will be elevated, and the difence between the two will be reproduced by about onehalf (2°C). The elevation in temperature inside the teste will be sufficient to stop spermatogenesis. Ther is no evidence that low ambient temperature will lower fertility.

The role of the scrotum and spermatic cord in temperature control of the testes involved drawing the testes closer swing further away from the body as amsient temperature rises. Two smooth muscles are involved. The tunica darttos, the smooth the spermatic cord, are sensitive to temperature. During cold weather, contraction of these muscles causes the scrotum to pucker and the spermatic cords to shorten, drawing the testes closer to the body. During hot weather, these muscles relax, peritting the scrotum to stetch and the spermatic cord to lengthen. Thus, the testes swing down away from the body These muscles do not rsepond to changes in temperature until near the age of puberty. They must be sensitized by testosterone to respond to changing ambient temperature.

Actual cooling of testes occurs by two mechanisms. The skin of the scrotum has both sweat abd sebaceous glands which are more active during hot weather. Evaporation of the secretions of these glands cools the scrotum and thus the testes. The external scrotum has been obsered to be 2°C to 5°C cooler than the temperature inside the testes. As the scrotum stretches during hot weather, more surface area is provided for cooling by evaporation. In addition to cooling occurs through heat exchange in the circulatory system. As arteries transproting blood at internal body temperature transcend the spermatic cord, their convoluted folds pass through a network of veins, the pampiniform venous plexus, transporting cooler blood back towards the heart. some cooling of arterial blood then occurs before it reaches the testes. The lengthening of the cord during hot weather provides more surface area for this heat exchange.

Epididymis

The Epididymis, the first external duct leading from the testis, is fused longitudinally to the surface of the testis and is encased in the tunica vaginalis with the testis and is encased in the tunica vaginalis with the testis. The single convoluted duct is coverd with an extensionof the tunica albuginea testis. The captut (head)of the epididymis is a flattened area at the apex of the testis, where 12 to 15 small ducts, the vasa efferentia, merge into a single duct. The corpus(body) extenging along the longitudinal axis of the testis is a single duct which becomes continuous with the cauda(tail). The total length of this convoluted duct is about 34 meters in the bull and longer in the ram, boar, and stallion. The lumen of the cauda is wider than the lumen of the corpus. The structure of the epididymis and other external ducts (vas deferens and urethra is similar to that of the tubular portion of the female tract. The tunica serosa (outer layer)is followed by a smooth muscle layer (middle)and an epithelial layer(innermost).

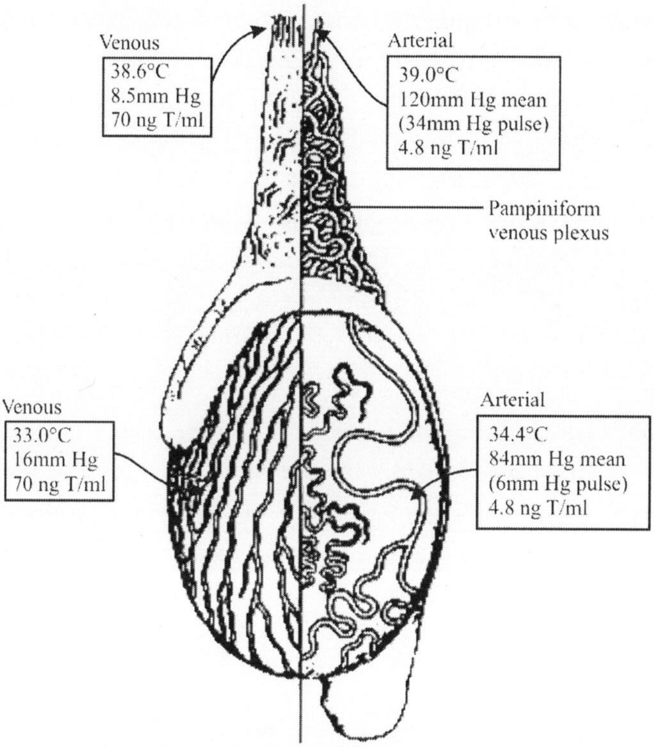

Fig. 16.6 Cooling of the Testis by Heat Exchange Through the Circulatory System.

(Setchell. 1977. Reproduction in Domestic Animals. (3rd ed) ed. Cole and Cupps. Academic Press

Transport

As a duct leading from the testes, the epididymis serves to transport spermatozoa. In sexually active males the time involved in transprot is 9 to 1 days in boars, 13 to 15 days in rams, and 9 to 11 days inbulls. Frequent ejaculation has been reported to speed transport by 10 to 20%.

Several factor contribute to movement of spermatozoa thorugh the epididymis. One factor is pressure from the production of new spermatozoa. As spermatozoa are produced in the seminiferous tubules, they are forced out through the rete testis and vasa efferentia into the epididymis. In a sexually inactive male, they are eventually forced through the epididymis. such movement of spermatozoa is aided by external perssure created by the massaging effect on the testes and epididymis thet occurs during normal exercise. The lining of the epididymis contains some ciliated epithelial cells, but the role of these cilia in facilitating movement of spermatozoa is aided by ejaculation. During ejaculation, peristaltic contractions involving the smooth muscle layer of the epididymis and a slight negative pressure (sucking action) created by peristaltic contractions of the vas deferens and urethra actively move spermatozoa from the epididymis into the vas deferens and urethra.

CONCENTRATION

A second function of the epididumis is concentration of spermatozoa. spermatozoa entering the epidiaymis from the testis of the bull, ram, and the epididymis, they concentrate to about 4x109(4 billion)spermatozoa per ml. Concentration occurs as the fluids, which suspend spermatozoa in the testes, are absorbed by the epithelial cells of the epididymis. Absorption of these fluids principally in the caput and proximal end of the corpus.

Storage

A third functin of the epididymis is storage of spermatozoa. Most are stored in the cauda of the epididymis where concentrated spermatozoa are packed into the wide lumen. The epididymis of a mature bull may contain 50 to 74 billion sperm. Capacities of other species are not reported. conditions are optimum in the cauda for preserving the viability of spermatozoa for an extended period. The low pH, high viscosity, high carbon dioside concentration, high potassium-to-sodium ratio, the influence of testosterone, and probably other factors combine to conteibute to a lower metabolic rate and extended life. These conditions have not been duplicated outside the epididymis. If the epididymis is ligated to prevent entry of new spermatozoa and removal of old, spermatozoa have remained have alive and fertile for about 60 days. On the other hand, after a long period of sexual rest, the first fewejaculates may contain a high percentage of nonfertile spermatozoa.

Maturation

A fourth function of the epididymis is that of maturation of spermatozoa. When recently formed spermatozoa enter the caput from the vasa efferentia they the ability for neither motility nor fertility. As they passthrough the epididymis they sain the ability to be both motile and fertile. If the cauda is ligated at each end, those spermatozoa closet to the corpusincreased in fertility for up to 25 days. During the same period, those closest to the vasa deferens exhibited reduced fetilizing ability. Therefore, it appears that spermatozoa gain ability to be fertile in the cauda and then start to age and deteriorate if they are not removed.

While in the epididymis, spermatozoa lose the cytoplasmic droplet which forms on the neck of each spermatozoa during spermatogenesis. The physiological significance of the cytoplasmic droplet is not known, but it has been used as an indicator of sufficient maturation of spermatozoa in the epididymis. If a high percentage of spermatozoa in fershly ejaculated semen has cytoplasmic droplets, they are considered immature and have low fertilizing capacity.

Vas Deferens and Urethra

The vas deferens are a pair of ducts with one leading from the distal end of the cauda of each epidymis. Initially supported by folds of the peritoneum, it passes along the spermatic cord, through the inguinal cannal to the pelvic region, where it merges with the urethra at its origin near the opening to the bladder. The enlarged end of the vas deferens near the urethra is the ampulla. The vas deferens has a thick layer of smooth muscles in its walls and appears to have single function of traspor of spermatozoa. Some have suggested that ampulllae serve as a short0term storage depot for semen. However, spermatozoa age quickly in the ampullae. It seems more likely that spermatozoa may pool in the ampullae during ejacualtion before being expelled into the urethra.

The urethra is a single duct which extends from the junction of the ampullae tothe end of the penis. It serves as an excretory duct for both urine and semen. During ejacualtion in bull and ram there is a complete mixing of spermatozoa concentrate from the vas deferens and epididymis with fluids from the accessory and boars, mixing is not as complete, with the ejaculate containing sperm-free and sperm-rich segments.

Accessory Glands

The accessory glands are located along the pelvic portion of the urethra, with ducts which empty their secretions into the urethra. They include the vesicular glands, the prostate gland and the bulbourethral glands. They contribute greatly to the fluid volume of semen. In addition, their secretions are solution of bufers, nutrients, and other substances needed to assure optium motility and fertility of semen.

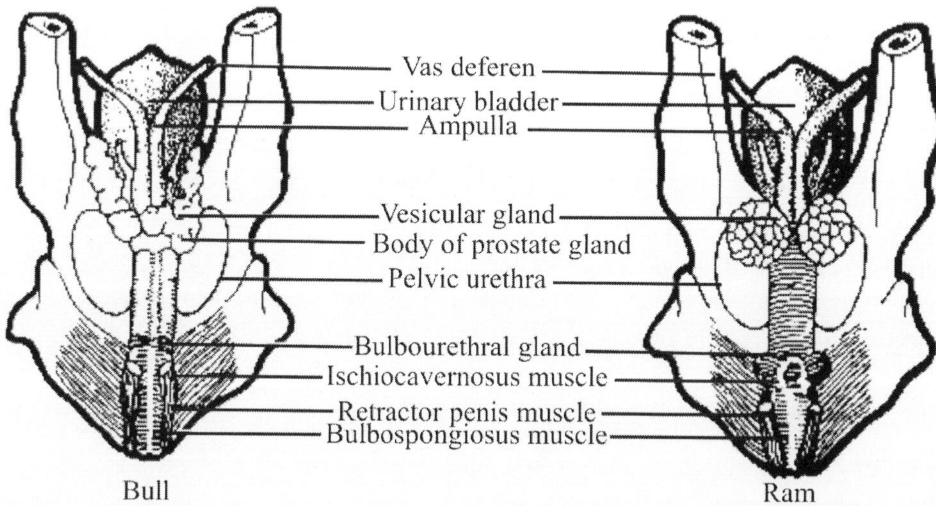

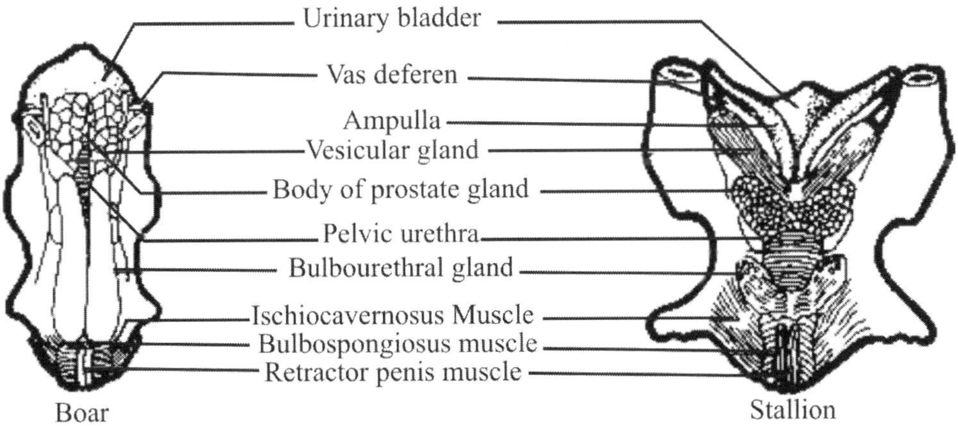

Fig. 16.7 a b Accessory Glands of the Bull, Boar, Ram, and Stallion Showing their Relationship to the Ampulla and Urethra. (Redrawn from Ashdown and Hancock. 1974. Reproduction in Farm Animals. (3rd ed). ed. Hafez. Lea and Febiger.)

VESICULAR GLANDS

The vesicular glands (sometimes called seminal vasicles) are a pair of lobular glands that are easily that identiied because of their knobby appearance. They have been described as having the appearance of a "cluster of grapes. " They are of similar length in the bull, boar, and stallion (35 to 15 cm), but the width and thickness of the vesicular glands of the bull is approxomately half that of the boar and stallion. They vesicular glands of the ram and buck are much smaller, being about 4 cm in length. The excretory ducts of the vesicular gkands open near the bifurcation where the ampullae merge with the urethra. In bulls, they contribute well over half of the total fluid volume of semen, and appear to make a substantial contribution in other species. Several organic compounds found in secretion of the vesicular glands are unique in that they are not found in substantial quantities elsewhere in the body. Two of these compounds, fruetose and sorbitol, are major sources of energy for bull and ram spermatozoa but are found in lower concentration in boar and stallion. Both phosphate and carbonate buffers are found in these secretions and are important in that they protect against shifts in the pH of semen. Such shifts in pH would be detrimental to spermatozoa.

Prostate Gland

The prostate is a single gland located around and along the urethra just posterior to the excretory ducts of the vesicular glands. A prostate body is visible in excised tracts and can be palpated in bulls and stallions. In rams, all of the prostate is embedded in urethra muscles as is part of this glandular tissue in bulls and boars. It makes a small contribution to the fluid volume of semen in mosr species stuided. however, some repory that the contribution of the prostate gland is at least as substatial as thet of the vesicular glands in boars. The prostate of the boar is larger than that of the bull. The secretions of the prostate are high in inorganic ions with sodium, chlorine, calcium, and magnesium all in solution.

Bulbourethral Glands

The bulbourethral (Cowpers) glands are a pair of glands located along the urethra near the point where it exits from the pelvis. They are about the size and shape of wanuts in bulls, but are much larger in boars. In bulls, they are embeded in the bulbospongiosum muscle. They contribute very little to the fluid volume of semen. In bulls, their secretions flush urineresidue from the urethra before ejaculation. These secretions are seen as dribblings from the prepuce just before copulation. In boars, their secretions account for that portion of boar semesn which coagulates. This strained from boar semen before it is used for artificial insemination. During natural service, the white lumps formed by coagulation may prevent semen from flowing bak through the cervix into the vagina of sows.

The Penis

The penis consists of connective tissue with numerous small blood spaces in it. These fill with blood during sexual excitement causing erection.

Dogs, bears, seals, bats and rodents have a special bone in the penis which helps maintain the erection. In some animals (e. g. the bull, ram and boar) the penis has an "S" shaped bend that allows it to fold up when not in use. In many animals the shape of the penis is adapted to match that of the vagina. For example, the boar has a corkscrew shaped penis, there is a pronounced twist in bulls' and it is forked in marsupials like the opossum. Some have spines, warts or hooks on them to help keep them in the vagina and copulation may be extended to help retain the semen in the female system. Mating can last up to three hours in minks, and dogs may "knot" or "tie" during mating and can not separate until the erection has subsided.

The penixl is the organ of copulation in males. It forms dorsally around the urethra from the point where the urethra leaves the pelvis, with the external urethral orifice at the free end of the penis. Bulls, boars, and rams have a sigmoid flexure, an S-shaped bend in the penis which permits it to be retracted completely into the body. These three species and the stallion have retractor penis muscles, a pair of smooth muscles which will relax to permit extension of the penis and contract to draw the penis back into the body. These retractor penis muscles aries from the vertebrae in the coccygeal region and are fused to the ventral penis just anterior to the sigmoid flexure. The glans penis (Figure 2.8), which is the free end of the penis, is wwell supplied with sensory nerves and is homologous to the clitorisin the female In most species the penis is fibroelastic, containing small amounts of erectile tissue. The penis of stallions contains more erectile tissue is found in bulls, boars, bucks, rams.

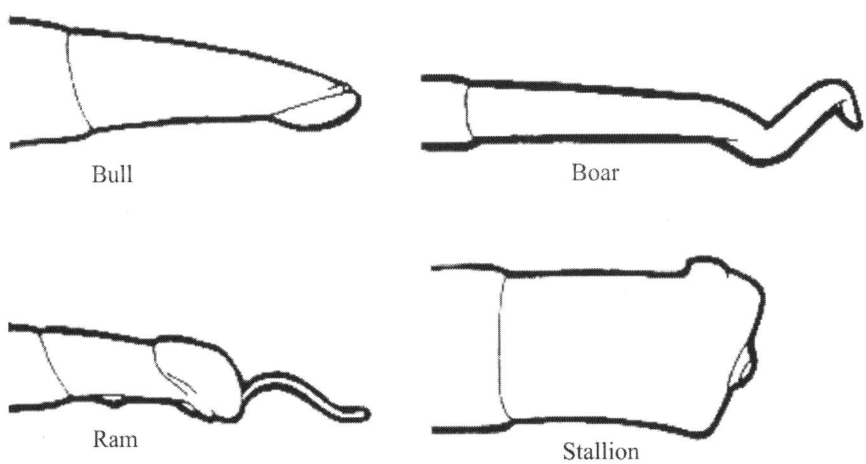

Fig. 16.8 a Comparative Diagram Showing the Shape of the Glans Penis of the Bull, Boar, Ram and Stallion. Note the Twisted Groove Containing the External Urethral Orifice in the Bull, the Urethral Proxess (filiform appendage) Extending beyond the Glands Penis ing the Ram, the Corkscrew Spiral in the Boar, and the Flattened Glans Penis in the Dtallion with the Small Urethral Process Extending Beyond. (Redrawn from Ashdown and Hancock. 1974. Reproduction in Farm Animals. (3rd ed.). ed. Hafez. Lea and Febiger.)

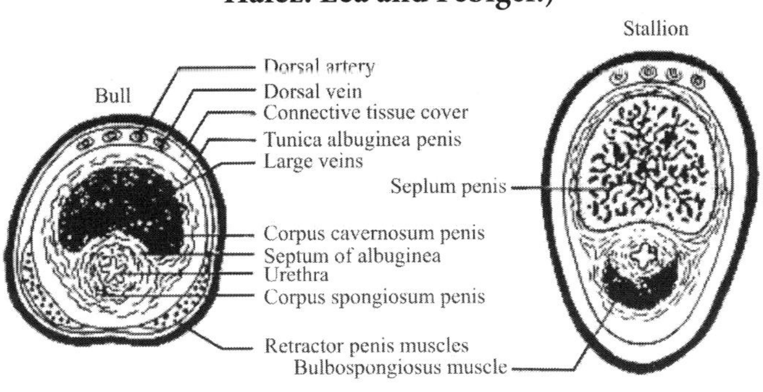

Fig. 16.8 b Cross Section of Penis Showing Corpus Cavernosum Penis and Corpus Spongiosum Penis. (Redrawn from Sprensen. 1979. Animal Reproduction: Principles and Practices. McGraw-Hill)

Erectile tissue is cavernous (spongy)tissue located in two regions of the penis. The corpus spongiosum penis is the cavernous tissue around the urethra. It enlarges into the penile bulb, which is cavered with bulbospongiosum muscle at the base of the penis. The corpus cavernosumpenis is a larger area of cavernous rods from the ischiocavernosus muscole , eventually fusing to from one cavernous area as it proceeds toward excitement, causing extension of the penis (erecrion)and facilitating the final ejection of semen during ejaculation. Both the bulbospongiosum muscle and ischiocavernous muscle are striated, skeletal muscles, rather than the smooth muscle associated with most of the male and female tracts.

Prepuce

The prepuce (sheath)is an invagination of skin which completely enclosed the free end of the penis. It has the same embryonic origin as the labia minora in the female. It can be divided into a prepenile portion, which is the outer fold, and the penile portion, or inner folds. The orifice of the prepuce is surrounded by long and tough preputial hairs.

Sperm

Sperm are made up of three parts: a head consisting mainly of the nucleus, a midpiece containing many mitochondria to provide the energy and a tail that provides propulsion.

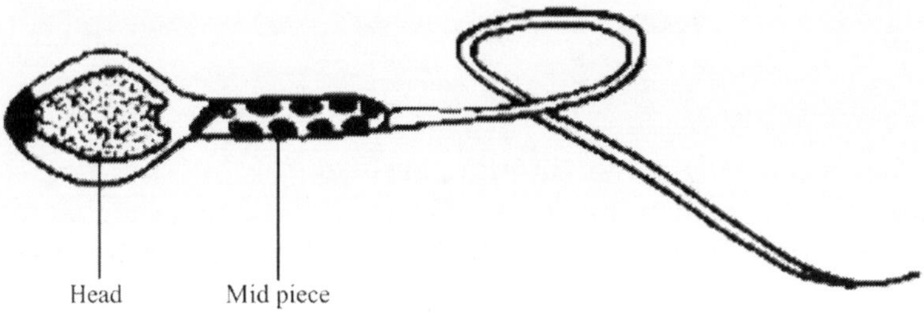

Fig. 16.9. A Sperm

A single ejaculation may contain 2-3 hundred million sperm but even in normal semen as many as 10% of these sperm may be abnormal and infertile. Some may be dead while others are inactive or deformed with double, giant or small heads or tails that are coiled or absent altogether.

When there are too many abnormal sperm or when the sperm concentration is low, the semen may not be able to fertilize an egg and the animal is infertile. Make sure you don't confuse infertility with impotence, which is the inability to copulate successfully.

Sperm do not live forever. They have a definite life span that varies from species to species. They survive for between 20 days (guinea pig) to 60 days (bull) in the epididymis but once ejaculated into the female tract they only live from 12 to 48 hours. When semen is used for artificial insemination, storage under the right conditions can extend the life span of some species.

ARTIFICIAL INSEMINATION

In many species the male can be artificially stimulated to ejaculate and the semen collected. It can then be diluted, stored and used to inseminate females. For example bull semen can be diluted and stored for up to 3 weeks at room temperature. If mixed with an antifreeze solution and stored in "straws" in liquid nitrogen at minus 79°C it will keep for much longer. Unfortunately the semen of chickens, stallions and boars can only be stored for up to 2 days.

Dilution of the semen means that one male can be used to fertilise many more females than would occur under natural conditions. There are also advantages in the male and female not having to make physical contact. It means that owners of females do not have to buy expensive males and the possibility of transmitting sexually transmitted diseases is reduced. Routine examination of the semen for sperm concentration, quality and activity allows only the highest quality semen to be used so a high success rate is ensured.

Since the lifespan of sperm in the female tract is so short and ova only survive from 8 to 10 hours the timing of the artificial insemination is critical. Successful conception depends upon detecting the time that the animal is "on heat" and when ovulation occurs.

Reproductive Anatomy and Physiology of the Bull

Good reproductive performance of a bull is necessary to obtain a high percent calf crop when natural service is used for breeding. A bull must be fertile, capable and willing to mate a large number of cows during a short breeding season for optimum production. A basic knowledge of the reproductive tract is beneficial for improved management. An understanding of the bull's reproductive system will also help the producer better understand breeding soundness examinations, reproductive problems and breeding impairments.

Anatomy

The reproductive tract of the bull consists of the testicles, secondary sex organs, and three accessory sex glands. These organs work in concert for formation, maturation and transport of spermatozoa, which are eventually deposited in the female reproductive tract. The secondary sex organs are the epididymis, vas deferens and penis. The three accessory sex glands include the seminal vesicles, prostate and bulbourethral gland (Cowper's gland).

Testicle

The testicle is located outside the body cavity in the scrotum and has two vital functions: producing the spermatozoa, and producing the male hormone, testosterone. Location of the testicles exterior to the body cavity is essential for normal sperm formation, which occurs only at 4 degrees to 5 degrees below body temperature. The scrotum provides physical protection to the testicle and helps regulate the temperature for optimum spermatozoa development. This regulation is done by coordination of three structures: a temperature-sensitive layer of muscle (tunica dartos) located in the walls of the scrotum, which relaxes when hot and contracts when cold; the external cremaster muscle within the spermatic cord, which controls the proximity of the testicle to the body by lengthening or shortening depending on environmental temperature; and a counter-current temperature exchange regulated by a blood flow process known as the pampiniform plexus, which is a coil of testicular veins that provide an effective mechanism for cooling arterial blood entering the testicle and transferring its heat to the venous blood leaving the testicle.

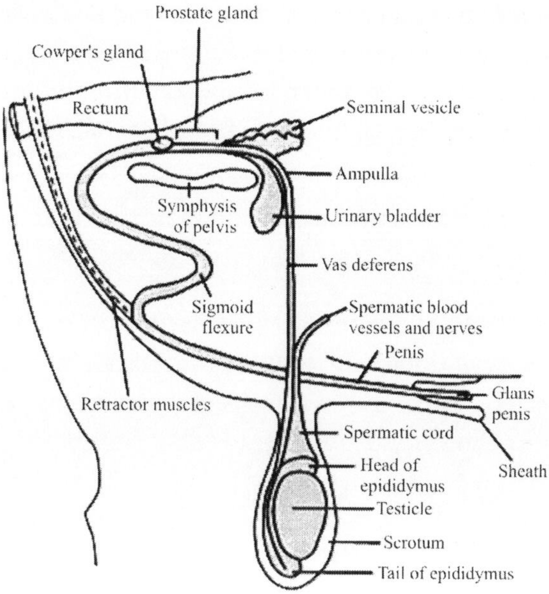

Fig. 16.10 Drawing of the Reproductive Tract of the Bull (from Nebraska Guide G80-536)

One or both testicles occasionally fail to descend into the scrotum during embryological development and are retained in the body cavity. This condition is known as chryptorchidism. Hormone production by chryptorchid males is near normal and the male develops and behaves like a normal male, but will generally be subfertile. This condition is genetically inherited, therefore such males should not be used for breeding.

The testicle contains many long, tiny, coiled tubes known as seminiferous tubules, within which the sperm are formed and begin to mature. Scattered throughout the loose connective tissue surrounding the seminiferous tubules are many highly specialized cells, the interstitial cells of Leydig, that produce testosterone. There are hundreds of individual seminiferous tubules in the body of the testicle which unite with one another to form a few dozen tubules that exit from the testicle and pass into the epididymis.

Epididymis

The epididymis is a compact, flat, elongated structure closely attached to one side of the testicle. It is divided into three regions, the head, body and tail. The many tubules entered the head of the epididymis from the testicle unite to form a single tubule some 130 to 160 feet in length. This tubule is convoluted and packed into the 6- to 8-inch epididymis. Four major functions occur in the epididymis, including the transport of the developing sperm cells from the testicle to the vas deferens; the concentration of the sperm by absorption of surplus fluids; the maturation of the developing spermatozoa; and the storage of viable sperm cells in the epididymis tail. If sexual activity is slowed, resorption of sperm cells from the epididymis tail occurs.

The epididymis serves as an outlet for all the sperm produced in the testicle and any blockage of this tube will cause sterility. Temporary blockage due to swelling following an injury or infection (epididymitis) will result in short-term infertility. If the swelling or infection results in formation of scar tissue in the tubule, it may permanently block the passage of sperm. If blockage occurs in both epididymides, the bull will no longer be useful as a breeder. Surgical removal of the tail of the epididymis (epididectomy) is frequently used as a means of sterilization for teaser (Gomer) bulls for estrus detection. Epididectomized bulls will still service cows in the usual manner, but will not deposit sperm in the female reproductive tract.

Vas Deferens

The vas deferens, also known as ductus deferens, emerges from the tail of the epididymis as a straight tubule and passes as part of the spermatic cord through the inguinal ring into the body cavity. Spermatozoa are transported further along the reproductive tract to the pelvic region through the vas deferens by contraction of the smooth muscle tissue surrounding this tubule during ejaculation. Bulls may also be sterilized by a vasectomy in which a section of the vas deferens is removed so that sperm cannot pass to the outside of the body.

Urethra

The two vas deferens eventually unite into a single tube, the urethra, which is the channel passing through the penis. The urethra in the male serves as a common passageway for semen from the reproductive tract and urine from the urinary tract.

ACCESSORY GLANDS

Two of the accessory glands are found in the general region where the vas deferens unite to become the urethra. Secretions from these glands make up most of the liquid portion of the semen. In addition, the secretions activate the sperm to become motile. The seminal vesicles consist of two lobes about 4 to 5 inches long, each connected to the urethra by a duct. The prostate gland is located at the neck of the urinary bladder where it empties into the urethra. The prostate is relatively small in the bull, as compared to other species, and does not produce a very large volume secretion.

The third accessory gland, the Cowper's glands, are small, firm glands located on either side of the urethra. The clear secretion that often drips from the penis during sexual excitement prior to service is largely produced by these glands and serves to flush and cleanse the urethra of any urine residue that may be harmful to spermatozoa.

One of the accessory glands may occasionally become infected, resulting in semen samples that are yellow and cloudy and which contain puss cells. It is not uncommon in bulls for the seminal vesicles to be so affected (seminal vesiculitis). Antibiotic treatment is sometimes necessary, but time will generally correct the problem.

Penis

The sigmoid flexure is an anatomical structure that provides a means by which the penis is held inside the sheath except during time of service. Strong retractor muscles hold the penis in the "S" shaped configuration. Occasionally these muscles are too weak to function properly and a portion of the penis and sheath lining protrude at all times. This exposes the male to the danger of injury and this characteristic should be avoided when selecting a herd bull.

The penis is the organ of insemination. Spongy-type material within the penis is filled with blood during sexual arousal, resulting in erection of the organ. The end of the penis is the glans penis and is richly supplied nerves, which are stimulated during copulation to induce ejaculation. Impairments of the glans penis may exist and should be detected during a fertility exam.

Regulation of Nale Hormones

The normal functions of male reproduction are largely controlled by hormones that are secreted from the endocrine glands. The testicle functions as an endocrine gland because of its production of the male hormone, testosterone, by the intersticial cells. Testosterone has several major functions:

- It is largely responsible for development and maintenance of the male reproductive tract
- It causes the development and maintenance of the secondary sex characteristics associated with masculinity, such as the crest and heavily muscled shoulders of a bull
- It is a major factor in the normal sex drive and behavior of the male
- It increases muscular and skeletal growth
- It is essential for normal sperm formation.

The testicle is, in turn, under the influence of hormones produced by other glands in the body. The same gonadotropic hormones that regulate ovarian functions in the cow also regulate testicular functions in the bull. Luteinizing hormone (LH) and follicle stimulating hormone (FSH) appear to be misnamed as pertaining to male reproduction, yet carry out several important male functions.

LH and FSH are released from the pituitary gland and cause the testicle to secrete testosterone, which then acts on the germ cell lining of the seminiferous tubules to stimulate formation of primordial sperm cells. The maturation of spermatids into fully developed sperm cells requires the presence of FSH. Normal functioning of the male accessory glands requires testosterone.

Not only is hormone production of the testicle regulated by hormones released by the anterior pituitary, but the reverse is also true. The level of testosterone in the blood regulates the secretion of gonadotropic hormones from the anterior pituitary via a feedback system. A proper balance of all hormones is vital to successful reproductive functions.

Breeding Soundness Exams

An examination of bulls for breeding soundness before the breeding season can detect the majority of bulls which have obvious potential fertility problems. This examination should be performed by an experienced, trained person, usually a veterinarian. It should be pointed out here that a breeding soundness examination is simply a screening procedure to eliminate bulls that have a high possibility of being non-fertile. A "fertility test" is a misnomer since techniques presently available do not allow for accurate prediction of fertility. Results from an actual breeding season remain the only test of a bull's breeding ability. Guidelines for a breeding soundness examination include:

PHYSICAL EXAMINATION

The penis should be examined during electro-ejaculation or natural mating, in an erected, extended state. Potential problems of the penis may include hair rings, which restrict circulation, a persistent frenulum or adhesion, lacerations, growths, scar tissue, deviations, or a urethral fistula. Next the scrotum and testes should be palpated. The scrotum should be pendulous but well supported. The testes should be firm and uniform in size and shape. The internal sex organs should be palpated rectally to ensure proper development and size. Good vision and sound feet and legs should also be considered when evaluating a bull's physical abilities to breed.

Scrotal Circumference

Scrotal circumference gives an indication of a bull's ability to produce sperm and is related to younger age at puberty. Breeds differ somewhat as to scrotal circumference, but 32 centimeters is generally accepted as the minimum size for yearling bulls to be sound breeds.

Semen Evaluation

Four criteria are used to evaluate semen, i. e., volume, concentration, motility and morphology. Proper training is required to accurately evaluate semen. A scoring system for predicting potential breeding soundness of bulls as prepared by the Society for Theriogenology, which incorporates scrotal circumference, semen motility, and semen morphology.

Breeding soundness examinations presently do not include an evaluation of a bull's sexual drive or libido. Libido testing is time consuming and requires use of females in estrus and therefore is difficult to conduct on a large scale. Procedures are being investigated to better evaluate the willingness and desire of bulls to mate.

REPRODUCTIVE SYSTEM IN DOGS

In male dogs, there is no seasonal period of increased or decreased sexual activity. Rather, they can be stimulated at any time by nearby females that are in season (heat).

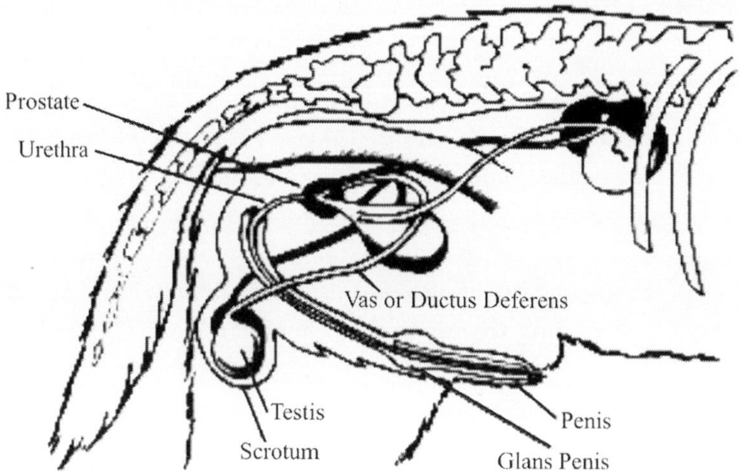

Fig. 16.11

In the male, the important structures of the reproductive system are the testicles, ductus or vas deferens, prostate gland, and penis. Sperm production and storage occurs within the testicles. Upon ejaculation, the sperm is transported to the prostate gland by the vas deferens. Within the prostate, additional fluids are added to the sperm to nourish it and aid in its transport from the penis and through the uterus.

The sperm and prostatic fluids, at the level of the prostate gland, enter the common urethra and are carried from the body through the penis. The penis of the dog has two specialized structures. The glans penis is a bulb-like dilation at the base of the penis, which fills with blood and holds the penis within the vagina during intercourse. Within the penis is a bone that maintains the shape and direction of this organ during mating. The penis is protected from the environment, as it is enclosed within the sheath or prepuce.

The more common disorders of the rMe productive tracts of puppies include vaginitis in females, and cryptorchidism and phimosis in males.

Female Reproductive System

The female reproductive system, consists of two ovarians and the female duct system. The duct system includes the oviducts, uterus, cervix, vagina, and vulva. The origin of the ovaries is the secondary sex cords of the genital ridge. The genital ridges are first seen in the embryo as a slight thickening near the kidneys. The duct system originates from the mullerian ducts, a pair ducts which appear during early embryonic development.

Ovaries

The ovaries are considered the primary reproductive organs in the female. They are primary because they produce the female gamete(the ovum) and the female sex hormones (estrogens and progestins). The cow, mare, and ewe are monotocous, normally giving birth to one young each gestation period. Therefore, one ovum is produced each estous cycle. The sow is polytocus, producing 10 to 25 ova each estrus cycle and giving birth to several young each gestation period.

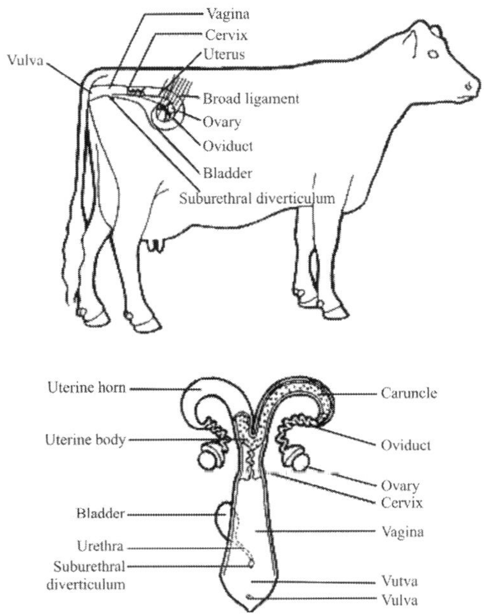

Fig. 16.12 Reproductive System and Associated Parts of the Urinary System of the Cow as it Appears in the Natural State (top) and Excised (bootom)

The ovary od the cow is described as almond-shaped, but the shape is altered by growing follicles or copora lutea. The average size is about 35×25×15mm. The size will among cows, and active ovaries are larger than inactive ovaries. Therfore, one ovary is frequently larger than the other in a given cow. The ovaries of the ewe and doe (goat) are almond-shaped and less than half the size of those of a cow. The ovaries in the mare are kidney-shaped and are two or three times larger than ovarie of a cow. The ovaries in the sow are slightly larger than those found in the ewe and appears as a "cluster of grapes".

The ovary is composed of the medulla and its outer shell, the cortex. The medulla is composed primary of blood vessel, nerves, and connective tissue. The cortex contains those cell and tissue layers associated with ovum and hormone production. The outermost layer of the cortex of the ovary is the surface epithelium. The surface epithelium because it was believed to be the odigin o female germ cells (oogonia). It is now known that germ cells do not arise from this epithelial layer. They aries from embryonic gut tissue and then migrate to the cortex of the embryonic gonad. Just beneath the sureace epithelium is a thin, dense layer of the connective tissue, the tunica albuginea ovarii. Bolow the tunica albuginea ovarii is the parenchyma, known as the functional because it contains ovarian follicles and the cells which produce ovarian hormones.

It is accepted that all primary follicle are formned during the prenatal period of the female. the greastest numbe are found in the fetal gilt 50 to 90 days postconception;the fetal calf 110 to 130 days postconception. A primary follical is agerm cell surrounded by a single layer of follicle (granulosa)cells. They are located in the oarencyma and are frequently seen in groups called egg nests. It is estimated that approximately 75, 000 primary follicles are found in the ovaries of a young calf. With continual follicular growth and maturation throughout her reproductive life, an old cew may have only 2500 potential ova. Some potential ova reach full maturity and are released into the duct system for possible fertilization and development of offspring. Most start development and become atretic (i. e., they degenerate). Therdore, the potential harvest of that could produce offspring is far greater than is actually realized.

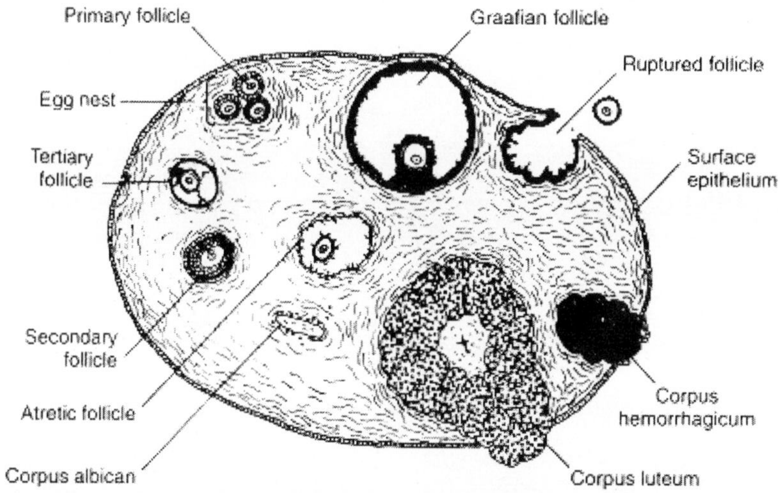

Fig. 16.13 Diagram of structures that can be identified in a cross section of an ovary of a reproductively active female. Different maturation stages for follicles and the corpus luteum can be observed. (Adapted from Patten. 1964. Foundations of Embryology. (2nd ed.) McGraw-Hill.)

Follicles are in a constant state of growth and maturation, A histological section of the cortex of a reprodictiovely active female will reveal these maturation stages. The primary follicle has been descrubed. This stage is followed by a proliferation of granulosa cells surroinding the potential ovum. A potential ovum surrounded by two or more layer of granulosa cells is secondary follicle. Later in the development, an antrum (cavity) will form by fluid collecting between the granulosa cells and seperating them. When the antrum has formed, the follicle is classified as a tertiary follicle. The mature tertiary follicle, which appears as a fluid-filled blister on the surface of the ovary, is also called a Graafian follicle.

The fluid in the antrum of a tertiary follicle is called liquor follicli. It is a viscous fluid that is rich in steroid reproductive hormones. particulary estrogens Recently a number of other reproductive hormones as well as nonhormonal factors that help regulate the function of the ovary have been identified in follicular fluid.

Several cell layers in the Graafian follicle have been identified and are of functional importance. The outer, more fibrous cell layer is the theca externa. Inside this layer is the theca interna. These two cell layers are supplied with blood by capillary network and can be differentiated microcopicaly with special histological staining techniques. Thecal cella and the capillay network are acquired as the follicle enlarges and pushes into the medulla. A basement membrane separates the theca interna from the innermost cell layer, the granulosa cells, and prevents entry of the vascular syatem into these cells(Figure 2-4). The granulosa cells surround the antrum. In addition, the cumulus oophorus, a hillock (mound)of granulosa cells, is located at one side of the antrum. The potential ovum rests upon the cumulus oophorus with other granulosa cells extending around the potential ovum. The granulosa cells surrounding and in immediate contact with the potential ovum are termed the corona radiata. Boththeca interna and granulosa cells are involved in production of estrogen. The theory is that the theca interna cells produce tetosterone, which diffuses through the basement membrane for conversion to estrogen by the granulosa cells. In addition, granulosa cells are the progesterone producing cells in the corpus luteum. They also secrete other compounds that have been identified infollicular fluid help regulate the function of the ovary. when ovulation occurs. the follicle ruptures expelling the liquor folliculi, some granulosa cells, and the potential ovum (oocyte)into the body cavity near the opending to the oviduct. At the time of expulsion, the oocyte is surounded by the corona radiata and a sticky mass containing other granulosa(cumulus) cells which aid the oviduct in picking up the oocyte and moving it down the oviduct. In some species the corona radiata is present at the time of fertilizition. In other species these cells are shed quickly and are not present when fertilization occurs.

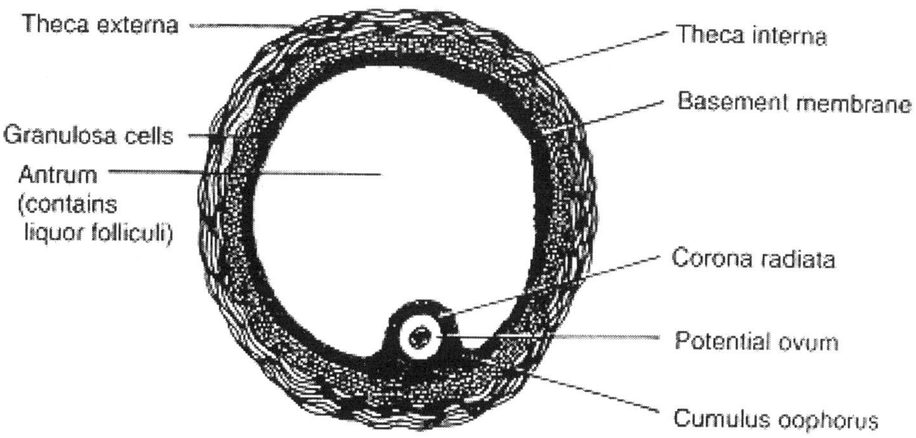

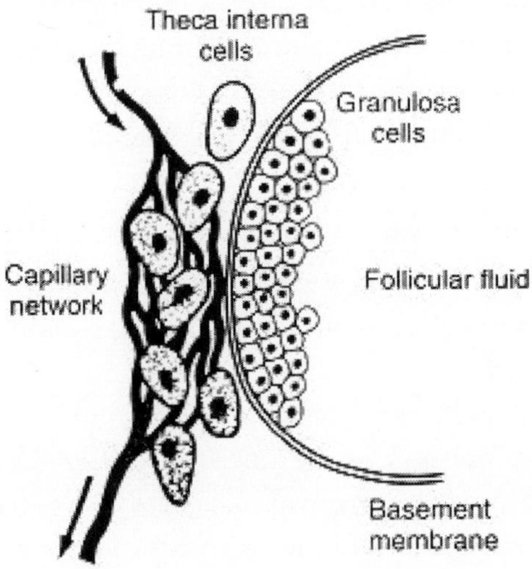

Fig. 16. 14. a,b Functionally important features of a Graafian follicle, (Redrawn from Hafez. 1974. Reproduction in Farm Animals. (3rd ed.) Lea and Febiger.)

Figure Structure of the wall of the Graafian follicle showing how the granulosa cells are deprived of a blood supply by the basement membrane. (Austin and Short. 1972. Reproduction in Mammals. 3. Hormones of Reproduction. Cambridge University Press.)

With rupture of the follicle, bleeding occurs and a blood clot forms at the ovulation site. The ruptured follicle with its blood-filled cavity is called a corpus hemorrhagicum. The corpus hemorrhagicum is replaced by the corpus luteum, which forms rapidly by proliferation of a mixture of theca externa, theca interna, and granulosa cells. Granulosa cells, which form the main component of the corpus luteum, enlarge and acquire a large amount of mitochondria and other intracellular structure involved in synthesis and secretion of progesterone. The corpus luteum is a solid, yellowish body which only ovarian source of these progestins. In a Holstein heifer between 1 and 4 days of the cycle, the average diameter of the corpus luteum is 8mm. Between 5 and 9 days, it has grown to an average of 15mm. The average maximum size of 20. 5mm is reached in 15 or 16 days in a heifer that is not pregnant. It then regresses in size with an average diameter of 12. 5 mm at 18 to 21 days. When the corpus luteum regresses, it no longer produces progestins. It loss its yellowish color, eventually appearing as a small white scar on the surface of the ovary, which is called a corpus albican. If the animal is pregnant, the corpus luteum will not regress until late pregnancy for most species, but species differences do exist

Oviducts

The oviducts (also called fallopian tubes) are a pair of convoluted tubes extending from near the ovaries to and becoming continuous with the tips of the uterine horns. Their functions include of ova and spermatozoa, which must be conveyed in opposite directions. In addition they are the site of fertilization and the early cell divisions of the embryo. Histologically, they contain three distinct cell layers. The outer layer, basically connective tissue, is the tunica serosa. The middle layer, composed of both circular and longitudinal smooth muscle fibers, is the tunica muscularies. The innermost layer, Which contains both ciliated and secretory epithelial cells, is the tunica mucosa. The same basic histological arrangement is found in the remainder of the female duct system with some differences in the inner two layers, which will be noted which be noted when we discuss specific organs.

An cviduct, which is from 20 to 30 cm long for most farm species, is divided into three segments. The funnel-shaped opening near the ovaries is the infundibulum. In some species(cat, rabbit, mink, and others)the infundibulum forms a bursa around the ovary. In the cow, doe, ewe, sow, and mare the infundibulum is separate from the ovary. There are numerous folds in the mucosa, and mucosal cells in the infundibulum are ciliates. The ampuula, the middle segment, is from 3 to 5 mm in diameter and accounts for about hlaf of the total length of the oviduct. The mocosal lining of the ampulla has from 20 to 40 longituidinal folds, which greatly increase the surface area of the lumen. The majority of the cells in the mucosa of the isthmus the third segment, at the ampullary-isthmic junction. This junction is difficult to locate anatomically and been descrubed as a physiological stricture which delay the ovum several is similar than the ampulla, being 0. 5 to 1 mm in diameter. It is further distinguished by having a thicker smooth muscle layer than the ampulla and from 4 to 8 mucosal folds. A higher ratio of secretory to ciliated cells is characteristic or the isthmus. The isthmus joins the tip of the uterine horn at the uterotubal junction. In general, oviductal activity is stimulated by estrogens and inhibited by progestins.

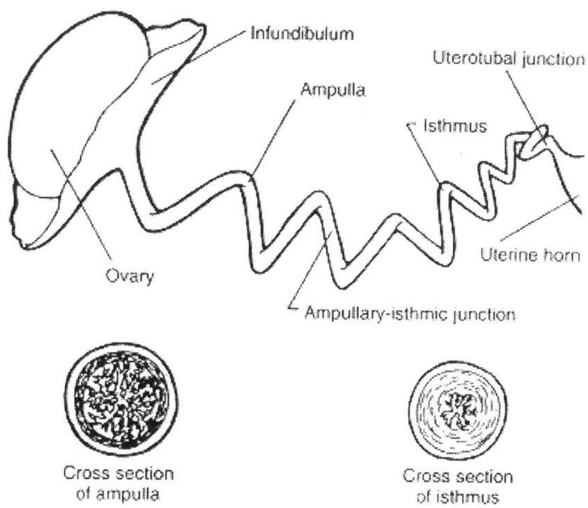

Fig. 16.15 Anatomy of the oviduct:top, longitudinal view illustrating the macroscopic features of the oviduct; bottom, cross section of the ampulla and isthmus comparing the thickness of the musculature of the wall and the complexity of the mucosal folds.

Uterus

The uterus extends from the uterotubal junctions to the cervix. For the cow, sow, and mare the overalll length may range from 35 to 60 cm. For the sow, doe, ewe, and cow the uterine horns account for 80 to 90% of the total length, wjile in the mare the uterine account for about 50% of the toal length. The uteri of the ewe and doe are less than half the size of the other mentioned soecies. The major function of the uterus is to retain and nourish the embryo, or fetus. Before the embryo becomes atatched to the uterus, the nourishment comes from yolk within the embtyo or from uterine milk which is secreted by glands in the mucosal layer of the uterus. After attachment to the uterus, nutrients and waste products are conveyed between materal and embryonic, or fetal, blood by way of the placenta.

Four basic types of uteri are found in animals. Only two of these types are found in farm animals. The bicornuate uterus is found in the sow, cow, doe, and ewe. It is characterized by a small uterine body just anterior to the cervical canal and two long uterine horns. Fusion of the uterine horns of the cow and ewe near the uterine body gives the impression of a larger uterine body than actually exists and has exists and has sometimes resulted in their uteri being classified bipartite. The sow has longer uterine horns than the cow, and they may slighyly convoluted. The mare has a biparitite uterus. There is a prominent uterine body anterior to the cervical cannal and two uterine horns thet are not as long and distinct as in the bicornuate type. During pregnancy in mares, the fetal body extends into both horns, whereas the fetuses do not occupy the uterine body in the bicornate types. The duplex uterus, which consists of thwo uterine horns each with a separate cervical cannal which opens into the vagina, is found in the rat, rabbit, guinea pig, and other small animals. The simople uterus, a pear-shaped body with no uterine horns, is characteristic of humans and other primates.

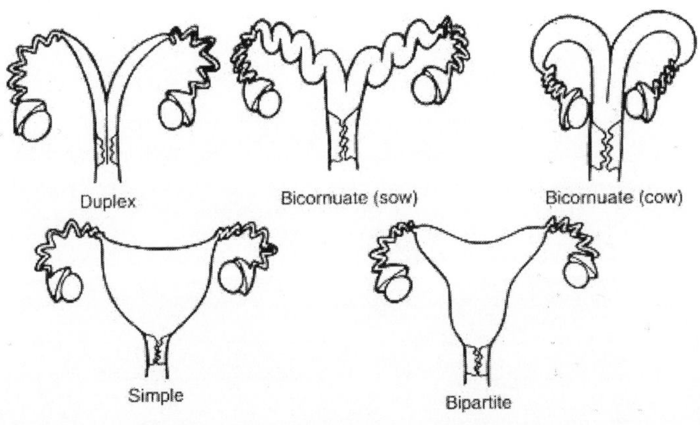

Fig. 16.16 Basic types of uteri found in mammals.

As in the oviduct, the tunica serosa is the outer layer of the uterus. The myometrium, the middle layer, is composed of two thin longitudinal layers of smooth muscle, with thicker cicular layer sandwiched between. estrogens increase the tone of the myometrium, causing the uterus to feelmore flaccid. The endometrium, the mucosal lining of the uterus, is more complex than the rest of the duct system and has simple glands. estrogens increase the vascularity and cause a thickening of the endometruim. in addition, estrogens stimulate growth of the endometrial glands. Progestins cause the emdometrial glands to coil and branch, and tosecrete uterine milk. The synergistic actions of estrogens and progestins on the endometrium are for preparation of the uterus of preganancy.

The endometrium provides a mechanism for attachment of the extraembryonic memberanes. This union forms the placenta, and the process is called placetation. With union forms the placeta, nutrients trom maternal blood can be transferred to embryonic or fetal blood and waste products from embryonic and fetal blood can be eliminated through the maternal systems. The nature of the placental attachment differs among soecied. cows, does, and ewes have cotyledonary placental attachments. Chorionic villi from the extraembryonic memberanes penetrate into caruncles, which are button-like projections on the endometirum. This union, chrionic villi and caruncle, forms the placentome (also called the cotyledon). There are 70 to 120 such cotyledonary attachments in a pregnant cow in late pregnancy. There are 88 to 96 in ewes and does, and these are smaller than in cows. The sow and , are have a diffuse (surface) placental ttachment. The extraembryonic membranes lie in folds on the endometrium, with chorionic villi ectending into the endometrium in more fragile attachment than is found in the cow, doe, or ewe.

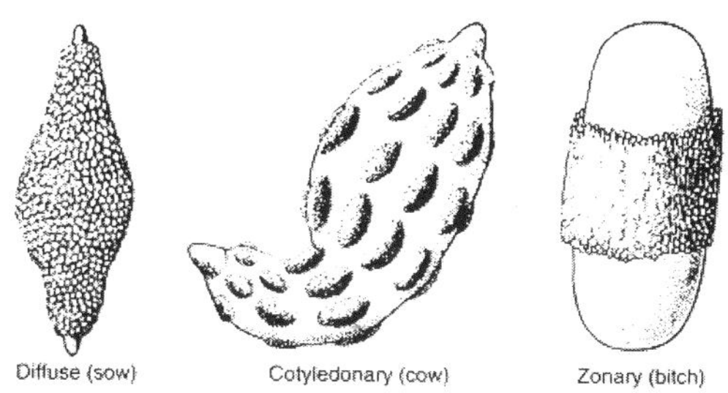

Figure 16.17 a Distribution of chorionic villi which serve as a basis of placental shape in several species. (Redrawn from Arey. 1974. Developmental Anatomy. (7th ed.) W. B. Saunders Co.)

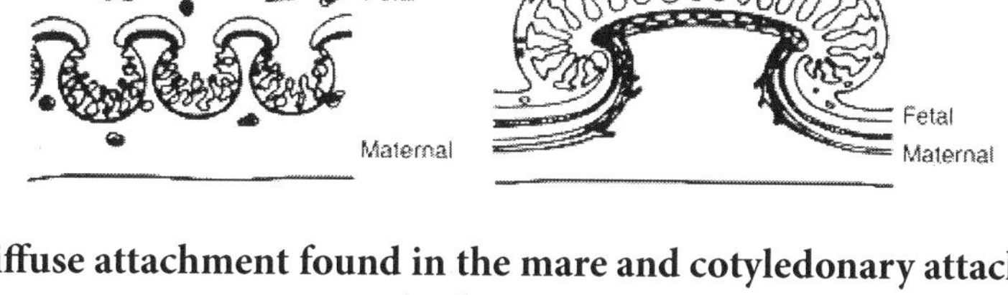

Fig. 16.17 b Diffuse attachment found in the mare and cotyledonary attachment found in the cow.

The placental attachment of the mare, sow, and cow is claasified as epitheliochorial. This means thartno erosin occurs either in the tissue of the extraembryonic tissue layer of the endometrium. formation of the placenta in the human results in rather extensive erosion of the endometrium. classified as hemochorial, nutients from maternal blood must pass through only extraembryonic tissues. Erosion is not extensive enough to result in direct mixing of materal and fetal blood in any mammalian species.

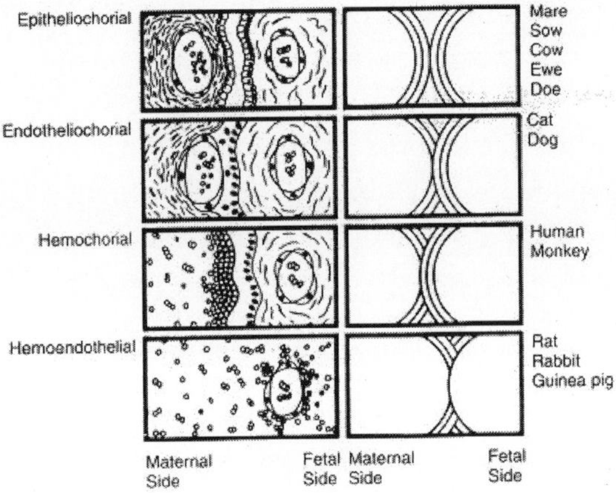

Fig. 16.18 Placental types showing the cellular barriers between maternal and fetal blood for several species. (Adapted from Arey. 1974. Developmental Anatomy. (7th. ed.) W. B. Saunders Co.)

CERVIX

While technically a part of the uterus, the cervix will be discussed as a distinct organ. It is thick-walled and inelastic, the anterior end being continuous with the body of the uterus while the posterior end protrudes into the vagina. For most farm species the length will range fron 5 to 10 cm with an outside diameter of 2 to 5 cm. It contains a canal which is the opening into the uterus. The primary function of the cervix is to prevent microbial contamination of the uterus;however, it also may serve as a sperm reservoir after mating. Semen is deposited into the cervix during natural mating in sows and mares.

The cervical cannals in the cow, doe, and ewe have transverse interlocking ridges known as annular rings which help seal the uterus from contaminants. The cervical cannal in the sow is funnel-shaped, with ridges in the cannal having a corkscrew configuration which conforms to that of the glands penis in the boar. The cervical cannal of the mare is more open than in other farm species, but mucosal folds in the canal which project into the vagina help prevent contamination.

Histologically, the outer layer of the cevix is the tunica serosa. The middle layer is connective tissue interspersed with smooth muscle fibers, whichgives the cervix its firm and inelastic properties. The inner layer, the mucosa, is composed mainly of secrectory epithelial cells, but some ciliated epithelial cells are present. High levels of estrogens cause the cervical canal to siliate during estrus (standing heat). Synergism between high levels of estrogens and relaxin causes greater dilation just before parturition. This dilation of the cannal would appear to make the uterus more vulnerable to invading organisms. However, estrogens cause the epithelial cells of the cervix to secrete mucus that antibacterial properties, thus protecting the uterus. If cervical mucus is obtained at estrus and allowed to dry on a glass slide, it will form a fern-like pattern. This ferning pattern does not form from cervical mucus obtained at stages of the cycle when estrogens are low. during pregnancy the mucus thickens into a gel-like plug, which seals and protects the uterus during the pregnancy. Removal of the mucus plug will increase the chance of abortion.

Vagina

The vagina is tubular in shape, thin-walled and quite elastic. It is from 25 to 30 cm in length in the cow and mare, and 10 to 15 cm in le ngth in the sow, doe, and ewe. In the cow, doe, and ewe, semen is deposited into the anterior end of the vagina, near the opening to the cervix, during natural mating. The vagina is the female organ of copulation.

The outer layer, the tunica serosa, is followed by a smooth muscle layer containing both circular and longitudinal fibers. In most species the mucosal layer is composed of startified squamous epithelial cells(the cow a possible exception). These epithelial cells cornify (become cells wothout nuclei) under the influence of estrugens. Vaginal smears can be used as an ai in detecting estrus, but are most useful in laboratory animals. This layer of cornified cells at the time of estrus may serve as a lubricating or protective mechaniasm which prevents abrasions during copulation. Under the influence of progestins, the epithelial lining regenerates.

BIBLIOGRAPHY

- Aspinall, Victoria; Cappello, Melanie; Bowden, Sally (2009), Introduction to Veterinary Anatomy and Physiology Textbook, Jeffery, Andrea (forward), Elsevier Health Sciences, ISBN 978-0-7020-2938-7
- Boden, Edward; West, Geoffrey Philip (1998), Black's veterinary dictionary, Rowman & Littlefield, ISBN 978-0-389-21017-7
- Done, Stanley H. (1996), Color atlas of veterinary anatomy: The dog & cat, Elsevier Health Sciences, ISBN 978-0-7234-2441-3
- Dyce, Keith M.; Sack, Wolfgang O.; Wensing, Cornelis Johannes Gerardus (2010), Textbook of veterinary anatomy, Saunders, ISBN 978-1-4160-6607-1
- Fenner, William R. (2000), Quick reference to veterinary medicine, John Wiley & Sons, ISBN 978-0-397-51608-7
- Lawhead, James B.; Baker, MeeCee (2009), Introduction to veterinary science, Cengage Learning, ISBN 978-1-4283-1225-8
- Pfeiffer, Dirk (2009), Veterinary Epidemiology: An Introduction, John Wiley and Sons, ISBN 978-1-4051-7694-1
- Radostits, O. M.; Gay, C. C.; Blood, D. C.; Arundel, J. H.; Hinchcliff, Kenneth W (2000), Veterinary Medicine: A Textbook of the Diseases of Cattle, Sheep, Pigs, Goats and Horses (9th ed.), Elsevier Health Sciences, p. 1877, ISBN 978-0-7020-2604-1
- Dunlop, Robert H.; Malbert, Charles-Henri (2004), Veterinary pathophysiology, Wiley-Blackwell, ISBN 978-0-8138-2826-8
- Eurell, Jo Ann Coers; Eurell, Jo Ann; Frappier, Brian L.; Dellman, Horst-Dieter (25 May 2006), Dellmann's textbook of veterinary histology, Wiley-Blackwell, ISBN 978-0-7817-4148-4
- Foreyt, William J.; Foreyt, Bill (2001), Veterinary parasitology reference manual, Wiley-Blackwell, ISBN 978-0-8138-2419-2
- Gupta, Ramesh Chandra (2007), Veterinary toxicology: basic and clinical principles, Academic Press, ISBN 978-0-12-370467-2

- Hirsh, Dwight C.; Maclachlan, Nigel James; Walker, Richard L. (2004), Veterinary microbiology, Wiley-Blackwell, ISBN 978-0-8138-0379-1
- Hunter, Pamela (2004), Veterinary Medicine: A Guide to Historical Sources, Ashgate Publishing, Ltd., p. 611, ISBN 978-0-7546-4053-0
- Merck, Melinda D. (2007), Veterinary forensics: animal cruelty investigations, John Wiley & Sons, ISBN 978-0-8138-1501-5
- Murphy, Frederick A. (1999), Veterinary virology, Academic Press, ISBN 978-0-12-511340-3
- Nicholas, Frank W. (2009), Introduction to Veterinary Genetics, John Wiley and Sons, ISBN 978-1-4051-6832-8
- Robinson, Wayne F.; Huxtable, Clive R. R. (2004), Clinicopathologic Principles for Veterinary Medicine, Cambridge University Press, p. 452, ISBN 978-0-521-54813-7
- Slatter, Douglas H. (2002), Textbook of small animal surgery, Elsevier Health Sciences, ISBN 978-0-7216-8607-3
- Kahn, Cynthia M., ed. (2010), The Merck Veterinary Manual, Whitehouse Station, N.J., Merck, ISBN 978-0-911910-93-3
- Thrusfield, Michael (2007), Veterinary epidemiology, Wiley-Blackwell, ISBN 978-1-4051-5627-1
- Zajac, A.; Conboy, Gary A.; American Association of Veterinary Parasitologists (2006), Veterinary clinical parasitology, John Wiley & Sons, ISBN 978-0-8138-1734-7
- Adams, H. Richard (2001), Veterinary pharmacology and therapeutics, Wiley-Blackwell, ISBN 978-0-8138-1743-9
- Bryant, Susan (2010), Anesthesia for Veterinary Technicians, John Wiley and Sons, ISBN 978-0-8138-0586-3
- Cannon, Marthaxcx; Hijfte, Myra Forster-van (2006), Feline medicine: a practical guide for veterinary nurses and technicians, Elsevier Health Sciences, ISBN 978-0-7506-8827-7
- Crispin, Sheila M. (2005), Notes on veterinary ophthalmology, Wiley-Blackwell, ISBN 978-0-632-06416-8
- Gelatt, Kirk N. (2000), Essentials of veterinary ophthalmology, Wiley-Blackwell, ISBN 978-0-683-30077-2

INDEX

R

S

T

U

V